UNSAFE PRACTICES
Restructuring and Privatization in Ontario Health Care

by Paul Leduc Browne

Canadian Centre for Policy Alternatives

Copyright © 2000 Canadian Centre for Policy Alternatives and the author.

All rights reserved. No part of this book may be reproduced or transmitted in any form or by any means, electronic or mechanical, including photocopying, or by any information storage or retrieval system, without permission in writing from the publisher or the author.

Canadian Cataloguing in Publication Data

Browne, Paul Leduc
    Unsafe practices: restructuring and privatization in Ontario health care

Includes bibliographical references
ISBN 0-88627-234-3

1. Health care reform—Ontario. 2. Medical policy—Ontario. 3. Privatization—Ontario. I. Canadian Centre for Policy Alternatives. II. Title.

RA395.C3B76 2000   362.1'09713   C00-901384-9

Printed and bound in Canada

Published by

Canadian Centre for Policy Alternatives
Suite 410, 75 Albert Street
Ottawa, ON K1P 5E7
Tel 613-563-1341   Fax 613-233-1458
http://www.policyalternatives.ca
info@policyalternatives.ca

Table of Contents

Table of contents iii

List of tables v

Acknowledgements vii

Preface 1

Chapter 1:
"Cascading Privatization": 1. Transforming the State 9
Health and health care are democratic rights 9
Health care, the market and the welfare state 10
De-commodification and privatization 12
How the privatization trend exploits
the internal crisis of health care 14
The wellspring of privatization in the Canadian state 15
The crisis of federal-provincial relations 17
The war on the poor 24
"Steering, not rowing"? Applying private-sector
management ideology to the public sector 25
The Harris government's agenda and the
neo-liberal managerial ideology 29
Ideological overlaps and ambiguities:
What does integration really mean? 31
Conclusion 36

Chapter 2
"Cascading Privatization":
2. The Impact on Health Care Services 37
Introduction 37
Cutting health care expenditures 38
Re-engineering health care 41
Slashing budgets and closing hospitals 43
Restructuring hospitals 49
"Rationalizing" the workforce 54
Private fund-raising 57

Long-term care 59
Ambulance services 64
User charges and de-insured services 68
Primary care 70
Conclusion 76

Chapter 3: Home Care 79
Introduction 79
Defining home care 81
Why care and costs are being shifted into the community sector 82
Home care is rationed 85
Re-engineering home care:
The introduction of managed competition 95
The impact of managed competition 117
Conclusion 130

Conclusion 133

Notes 141
Preface 141
Chapter 1 144
Chapter 2 153
Chapter 3 163
Conclusion 173

List of Tables

Table 1: Federal transfers to Ontario under
EPF and CHST, actual and estimated, 1991-2004 22

Table 2: Provincial government expenditures on health care in
millions of constant dollars, Ontario, 1994-2001 39

Table 3: Real private health care expenditures per capita 40

Table 4: Hospital beds in Ontario, 1989-1998, by year and category 44

Table 5: Number of cases discharged from Ontario hospitals,
by year and type of hospital, 1989-1998 (hospital separations) 45

Table 6: Provincial transfer payments for the
operation of hospitals, 1994-2001, Ontario 46

Table 7: Summary of hospital costs
resulting from HSRC directions, May 1999 48

Table 8: Projected 1998/1999 hospital deficits in Ontario 48

Table 9: Nursing jobs gained or lost between 1994 and 1999 54

Table 10: Provincial transfer payments for long-term-care
residential services, 1994-2001, in constant 2000 dollars 64

Table 11: Provincial government
expenditures on ambulances, 1994-2000 67

Table 12: Transfer payments made for services and care
provided by physicians and practitioners, 1995-2001 72

Table 13: Rate of increase of average CCAC professional
visits and homemaking hours, 1996-1999 89

Table 14: Provincial government expenditures on home
care in constant (2000) dollars and per program, 1994-2001 90

Table 15: Comparison of volume of homemaking hours and professional
visits with Ontario Ministry of Health Funding, 1996-1999 91

Table 16: Hamilton-Wentworth CCAC—
intended RFP schedule (March 2000) 104

Table 17: The balance between quality
and cost in CCACs' RFP Processes 105

Table 18: Provider agencies under contract with CCACs,
nursing, 1996-1999 119

Table 19: Provider agencies under contract with CCACs,
home support/homemaking, 1996-1999 120

Table 20: Provider agencies under contract with CCACs,
physiotherapy, speech pathology & social work, 1996-1999 122

Table 21: Provider agencies under contract with CCACs,
equipment and medical supplies, 1996-1999 122

Acknowledgements

Although I am of course solely responsible for the contents of this report, I could not have written it without the help of many others, who contributed advice, information and encouragement. It is not possible to thank them all here individually, but I wish to assure them of my appreciation.

I am particularly grateful to Pat and Hugh Armstrong for their tact, encouragement, constructive criticism and judicious suggestions. My colleagues at the Canadian Centre for Policy Alternatives, Bruce Campbell, Ed Finn, Kerri-Anne Finn, Diane Touchette, and Erika Shaker, were a constant source of help and advice. Donna Vogel lent me her ears and eyes at a crucial moment. John Loxley and Marc Lee gave valuable advice on the presentation of some of the research findings. Many thanks to Abdollah Omid Payrow Shabani, Phil Eles, and Ted Haines for their help in gathering data. I am grateful to Bill Murnighan, Mike McBane, Janet Maher, Cathy Robinson, Stan Marshall, Heather Farrow, Vanessa Kelly, Megan Park, Ross Sutherland, Colleen Fuller, and Hugh Mackenzie, for supplying me with valuable information, as well as to Andrea Gabber and M. Forbes at the Ontario Hospital Association and Kim Jarvi of the Registered Nurses Association of Ontario for their help. Susan Donaldson and many employees and executives of CCACs and provider agencies spoke with me, gave generously of their time, filled out questionnaires, and shared their knowledge. My warm thanks to them all. I would also like to express my appreciation to all the officials of the Ontario Ministry of Health and Long-Term Care and the Ontario Management Board Secretariat, as well as the federal Department of Finance, who provided me with information. Research for the home care chapter of this book was partly financed by the "Économie sociale, santé et bien-être" project co-ordinated by Daniel Labesse and Yves Vaillancourt and funded by Human Resources Development Canada's Social Partnership Program.

Lastly, and most importantly, I wish to thank Michelle Weinroth and Raphaël Weinroth-Browne for their patience, support and solidarity.

Preface

Medicare has often been described as Canada's most cherished social program. It is not hard to understand why. Its practical value is second to none. Of all the afflictions that human beings may suffer, those that directly affect their very bodies are both the most menacing and the most universal. Even when it does not threaten our very existence, illness disrupts the normal course of our lives; it may precipitate economic ruin and social isolation by making us unable to work. Medicare promises everyone access to relief and even a cure, without requiring direct payment in return and without distinction of age, gender or region of origin. Medicare has worked, and worked well for Canadians.

"I realized just how valuable medicare is the night I had to rush my three-year-old son to emergency at two o'clock in the morning," says Pierre B., a school teacher in Timmins, Ontario. "My son was immediately looked after, and no one asked us whether or how we would pay for the care. It gives us such a sense of security, knowing that health care is there whenever we need it."

At its best, medicare reflects all that is noblest and most efficient about the welfare state. It ensures that the universal risk of ill health is equitably shared by all, in effect transferring part of the economic burden of care from the unhealthy and "unwealthy" to the healthy and wealthy.[1] As a universal, accessible, comprehensive, portable, and publicly administered system, medicare is the strongest remaining pillar of the welfare state.[2] The others have either been discarded as public policy priorities (full employment, universal family allowances and old age pensions), or been gutted (unemployment insurance).

But medicare also holds such a deep appeal because it speaks so eloquently to our sense of identity. It is a story of communities emerging from war and a colonial past to build new institutions in their own image—and which reflect back to them a new, bolder image. Furthermore, it is a tale about how communities pulled together to triumph over sickness, death, and the power of money.[3] It has all the ingredients of a gripping epic. It's hardly surprising that it should appeal so to Canadians.

Today, Canadians are extremely worried about the future of medicare. Survey after survey shows that health care is the number one priority, far ahead of education, tax cuts, and even employment, long the issue of greatest concern. For example, in an Angus Reid poll conducted in December 1999, 62 percent of respondents ranked health care as the main priority for the government, 49 percent felt education was the most important issue, and 25 percent pointed to poverty instead (respondents were allowed to cite two issues).[4] Overcrowded emergency rooms, nursing shortages, waiting lists for surgery, patients being sent to the United States for cancer care, skyrocketing costs——if daily media reports are true, Canada's health care system is breaking down. And while medicare remains enormously popular, opinion surveys indicate that most citizens are very worried about its viability. In the Angus Reid poll, 71 percent of respondents agreed with the statement that Ontario's health care system is in a crisis.

Efforts by the federal government to deflect and defuse such worries have failed. The announcement of increased health care funding in the 2000 federal budget was clearly meant to appease voters' fears; instead public anxiety has only become more inflamed.[5] The provincial premiers' reaction can only have thrown more fuel on the fire. They have repeatedly hinted that federal failure to transfer far greater sums to them for health care could result in drastic changes to the system, in particular privatization. Ontario Premier Mike Harris raised the spectre of user fees for health care.[6]

What is privatization? It is perhaps most often thought of as the sale of government assets, such as land or companies, to the private sector. But it can take many other forms as well. Privatization is a process whereby *activities, assets, costs, or control are shifted from the public to the for-profit private sector*. The latter, in other words, replaces the public sector in doing, owning, paying for, or controlling something. Such a shift may assume an "explicit and direct" or "implicit and indirect" form. The former includes:
- "disposing of state-owned assets, including land, infrastructure, and state-owned enterprises, through sales, leases, or liquidation" (transferring ownership);
- "substituting state-financed but privately produced services for state-produced services, as in contracting out, the distribution of vouchers, and other forms of payment for private provision."

The "implicit and indirect" forms of privatization are:
- "the disengagement of government from a sphere of service provision," either abruptly, so that citizens immediately have to purchase an equivalent in the marketplace, resort to charity, supply their own service, or do without—or slowly, by attrition, as governments gradually starve services of financial and other resources, encouraging citizens to look elsewhere for an alternative to deteriorating services;
- "the deregulation of entry into state-owned monopolies."[7]

Put another way, the privatization of public services occurs when governments:
- cease altogether from paying for a service or providing it;
- still pay for a service, but no longer deliver it themselves, or do so less, instead turning to the private for-profit sector to do so;
- still provide the service, but require someone else, such as the user, to assume part or all of the cost;
- still provide and pay for a service, but manage and deliver it along the lines of a commercial, for-profit enterprise.

Some of the key policies and policy instruments associated with privatization are service reductions, contracting out, public-private partnerships, cost shifting (user fees, de-listing, de-insuring), commercialization, and organizational restructuring.

Canada's health care sector is a mixed economy. The government pays for care by physicians and in hospitals, as well as for a range of related aspects of care. Individuals must pay for most dental care, prescription drugs, and a number of other items, privately. Most care has been delivered by independent professionals working on a fee-for-service basis, such as physicians, dentists, optometrists, psychiatrists, occupational therapists, physiotherapists, and midwives, or non-profit institutions, such as hospitals.[8] Private corporations supply drugs and medical equipment, operate some nursing homes, and so on.[9]

Privatization in the Canadian context means changing the composition of the mixed economy of health care at the levels of governance, financing, or service delivery.[10] Increasingly, for example, individuals are being asked to pay directly, or via private insurance, for at least a part of some services that used to be publicly insured, or are having to seek care from private, for-profit firms. For those without the money, this means doing without needed care, or relying more on the unpaid labour of family, friends and neighbours.

In general, the consequences of privatization are higher costs, diminished access, less efficiency, lower quality of care, and loss of public control over these vital services:

[H]ealth care is not a commodity like others. It does not benefit from market-based reforms. For-profit competition increases costs, drives up administrative efficiencies, creates barriers to equal access for all people, and can threaten quality of care. Private, for-profit health care has been proven conclusively to be a bad idea for almost everyone.[11]

Health-care privatization is very much in the headlines, as the Alberta government expands the role of private clinics in that province. The debate about the pros and cons of such a move rages across the country. The spectre of privatization is certainly very real in Ontario. The Harris government has long espoused an ideological commitment to privatization. And while it has promised not to weaken medicare, it has proclaimed its openness to outright privatization of public services in general, and its eagerness to promote so-called public-private partnerships. In a February 2000 speech, for example, Ontario Finance Minister Ernie Eves stated that his government would entertain any "reasonable" proposal from private corporations seeking "a financial stake" in public institutions and infrastructure: "Everything is on the table, every idea will be considered, every concept will be explored. If the private sector can find a way of providing services currently provided by the government in a way that is more cost-efficient and improves the quality of that service, then we are ready to listen."[12] Premier Mike Harris made similar remarks about health care in a speech the same month to a Progressive Conservative Party policy conference. Warning that health care costs are likely to escalate substantially, the premier "said one issue that needs to be discussed is to what extent people will be required to cover their own health-care costs. 'I can't answer that,' Mr. Harris said when asked how much people will be required to pay in the future. 'It may be that they'll pay for even less out of their own pockets.'"[13]

Influential voices around the Ontario government are calling very explicitly for privatization. Their common theme is that medicare is financially unsustainable, mainly because of the cost of new technology and the aging of Canada's population, and because Canada's national debt is too great to allow for deficit-financing. Some also claim that any public system is intrinsically likely to be inefficient and wasteful.[14]

Declaring that hospital funding will need to increase by 600 percent by 2004, the president of the Ontario Hospital Association told the Standing Committee on Finance and Economic Affairs of the Ontario Legislature that more private spending on health care will be needed in the future, because the public sector will not be able to meet the needs in an era of balanced budgets.[15] The Fraser Institute, a right-wing Vancouver organization with ties to the Ontario government, has long called for medicare, indeed most public services, to be supplanted by private market-based alternatives.[16] Member of Parliament Keith Martin, a leadership candidate for the Canadian Alliance, says that the shortage of money for medicare can be remedied by creating a parallel private health care system, entirely paid for with private money: "People accessing private services would no longer be draining the public system, thereby leaving more money and better care for those still in the public system. The private system would in effect be strengthening the public system."[17] (As if Mr. Martin's private system would not drain money, talent, resources, and political support away from the public system even more rapidly!)

This is very much at odds with public opinion. The December 1999 Angus Reid poll showed that 55 percent of Ontarians would favour raising taxes for health care, 66 percent rejected a two- tier health care system, and 65 percent were against putting "major limits on the healthcare services provided to Ontarians." The majority therefore seems clearly in favour of increasing public spending on health care, maintaining levels of service, and rejecting a two-tier system.[18]

Of course, statements by politicians, businessmen and advocacy groups are not in themselves proof that privatization really is occurring. However, analysis of government policy and spending shows that the balance is indeed tipping in that direction. To be sure, the Ontario government has not said or done anything to suggest that it will throw the hospital sector wide open to competition from private hospitals, nor has it said that doctors will be allowed to bill patients directly for all the services that are currently insured by the Ontario Health Insurance Plan. The Harris government has repeatedly expressed its support for the Canada Health Act. But privatization can take many roads and many years to arrive. Medicare is too popular in Canada for any government to challenge it openly.

It should be recalled that the huge cuts to social spending of the mid-1990s only came after the federal government and business interests had spent a decade changing Canadians attitudes with concerted and constant propaganda about the supposedly disastrous implications of the national debt[19] and a host of piecemeal changes to social programs (which Ken Battle referred to as "social policy by stealth"). Similarly, Ontario today is witnessing piecemeal privatization in health care: the introduction of private-sector business strategies and management ideologies into the public health care system; reductions and stagnation in public spending in the sector; the reduction, restructuring and rationing of publicly delivered services (especially hospitals); cost-shifting from the public purse to the individual household.

Privatization is not a one-off event, or even a number of isolated incidents, but a *process*. It amounts to much more than this or that specific government policy, decision by a hospital's board of directors, or action by a private corporation. Pat Armstrong has evoked the useful metaphor of a "cascade" to describe it. This is how the cascading effect looks:

The federal government adopts a neo-liberal policy framework, enters into "free-trade" agreements with other countries, and in the name of competition begins dismantling social programs to eliminate "labour-market rigidities" (i.e. to push down wages). As part of this process, it invokes its fiscal crisis, saying that the national debt is unsustainable and that public spending must be reduced. Federal transfer payments to the provinces (including for health care) are one of the main targets of the cuts.

The provincial governments themselves heartily embrace the neo-liberal or neo-conservative agenda. They too reduce transfer payments to lower levels of governments, slash social programs, rewrite labour legislation and regulations in favour of employers, and adopt private-sector managerial ideologies and practices, in the form of an "alternative service delivery" program.

Forced by the provincial government's cost-containment agenda to reduce their own spending, and driven by the same private-sector ideology, institutions and agencies adopt their own private-sector practices, such as total quality management. Health care and social services become less accessible, less affordable and of lesser quality.

Diminished quality and access are then used by neo-liberals as evidence that the public sector is inefficient and that further privatization is necessary. Meanwhile, those with money seek better quality and swifter access in the private sector. Abandoned by (at least part of) the middle class, the public system no longer garners universal support and becomes very weak politically.[20]

Chapter 1 tells of the first two waves in this cascade: (1) the federal government's reduction in transfer payments to Ontario; and (2) the Ontario government's neo-conservative agenda, its "alternative service delivery" ideology, and the equivocal wrapping—the integrated health system—in which this agenda has been sold and justified. Together, these are the story of privatization as the economic, political, ideological and administrative attack on Canada's social welfare state.

Chapter 2 follows the cascading movement through the different components of Ontario's health-care system: the Ministry of Health's overall spending envelope, hospital restructuring, the privatization of services, such as laboratory testing, the impact on the workforce, long-term institutional care, ambulance services and public health, new user charges, and primary care.

Chapter 3 takes a more in-depth look at the transformations taking place in home care in Ontario.

Although privatization policies and cutbacks at each level impel other governments and institutions to follow suit, it must be stressed that those other governments and institutions are also driven to do so by their own dominant interests and ideologies. Federal cutbacks have encouraged Ontario to slash spending and privatize—but the Ontario government would have done so anyway on the basis of its neo-liberal ideology and the powerful business interests it serves, as I shall explain in Chapter 1. Similarly, as we shall see in Chapter 2, hospitals have been compelled by the provincial government to restructure and reduce their operations and staff. But certain management trends within hospitals have tended in the same direction. In other words, there are internal and external forces working together and reinforcing each other at each level of the process to promote privatization.

None of which is to imply that these changes were inevitable. On the contrary, public policy is about *choices*. At each level, different choices could have been made.[21] To describe the trend that has been dominant is not to imply that it was the only one, or the only viable one. Indeed, at each level there are also citizens working to oppose privatization, either individually or through the associations, coalitions or unions to which they belong.[22]

The period studied here is 1995-2000. This should not be interpreted as an implicit statement that there was no privatization in health care in Ontario before 1995. Nor should it be thought that the intention was to single out the Conservative government for particular scrutiny or criticism. In many ways, the Harris government has walked on a path blazed by its predecessors. Had the resources available for the study been greater, it would have been fascinating and instructive to survey health care's evolution over a much longer period, certainly over the entire 1980s and 1990s. Unfortunately, that will have to await another book.

Chapter 1

"Cascading Privatization":
1. Transforming the State

This first chapter explains the context in which privatization is occurring and outlines the first moments of the cascade evoked by Pat Armstrong. I begin with a preliminary discussion of privatization, in which I outline some of the important values that it threatens, such as democracy and social rights. I then go on to explain some of the historical background to the current privatization movement: on the one hand, the crisis in federal-provincial relations, on the other hand the rise of Neo-Conservatism in Ontario. I follow this with a discussion of the Ontario Conservative government's vision of the public sector, and of public health care in particular. I conclude the chapter with some comments on the ideological contradictions at work behind integrated health delivery, a key notion in the debate over the future of health care in Ontario.

Health and health care are democratic rights

When Pierre B. of Timmins, Ontario, went to the hospital with his son at two o'clock in the morning, he was confident in his ability to receive care, because he expected it *as his right*. He knew that he was *entitled* to it as a *citizen* of Canada.

The right to health and to care is enshrined in Canadian law and in the covenants of the United Nations. It is a vitally important part of citizenship. It exemplifies the fact that we are all *equal*: each and every one of us has a right to be looked after, regardless of race, creed, or *ability to pay*. But is also helps *make* us equal: because everyone receives care when needed, we are all healthier, and therefore better off for it. We are all better able to take up our rightful places in society.

Having rights such as this *empowers us as citizens*. It is part and parcel of what gives each of us the authority to form his or her own opinions, to speak up, to participate in public life. It is a matter of *democracy*.

For our right to health and health care to be effective, to be genuine, *it is crucially important* that health care not be a commodity, that it not be left to the marketplace to provide. Being just another commodity would prevent it from being a right. Of course, we have a "right," in an abstract sense, to buy anything we please on the market, provided we can pay for it. Nobody forbids us from purchasing a Porsche. Hardly anyone exercises this "right," since only a few have the money to do so. But when we say that everyone has a right to health and health care, we mean something much stronger and deeper: we attach *no condition* to it, such as the ability to pay. Everyone has a right to health, period. Anyone who is ill has a right to care from a physician or in a hospital, period.

The right to health and to health care is at the very core of Canadian citizenship today. But it was not always so. To understand how it came to be and why it is under threat today, it is important to think about what *kind* of society Canada became during the three decades following the Second World War, and how it has been changing over the last twenty years.

Health care, the market and the welfare state

The Canadian state is embedded in a liberal market society, in which it plays two diametrically opposed roles. It creates and maintains conditions in which the free market and free enterprise can flourish, in order to generate the right climate for businesses to make profits. But it must also curb and regulate the free market, in order to cement social cohesion and ensure political stability.

Liberal economic theory says that, in order to nurture private business, the state establishes a legal and regulatory framework that protects property, rewards initiative, encourages competition, punishes corruption and violence, and allows the market to allocate resources by setting prices. According to this theory, taxation, public sector borrowing, and public measures to enhance health and welfare will be regarded as excessive if they interfere with the efficient allocation of resources by the market, for example by increasing the price of labour or capital (wages and interest). The classical liberal doctrine of laissez-faire should apply: let the market regulate society as much as possible, with minimal government intervention to keep order and make sure everyone plays by the rules.

However, left to its own devices, the market *fails* in various ways. It allows only for behaviour that yields profits for individual entrepreneurs. While curing disease may prove profitable, there is no profit to be made in its prevention—market-driven health care is entirely focused on curative rather than preventative medicine. Private health-care businesses also channel money away from care and into the pockets of shareholders.

The market cannot protect those who are unable to bargain for themselves, but leaves them at the mercy of unscrupulous businesses. This is why the market is widely held to produce inferior personal care services for children, elderly people or the very ill. Furthermore, a person living in a long-term care facility is really neither in a position to shop around and sample the different alternatives available, nor to move to another facility should the one she is in prove inadequate. In Ontario, there are waiting lists as long as three years to get into some long-term care facilities.

The market cannot address "externalities." For example, it may offer no incentives to entrepreneurs to provide services in areas that are geographically remote from urban centres or which have a low population density. A case in point is the situation in a rural part of Ontario, where the agency that brokers home care services on behalf of the provincial government has not been able to contract out certain therapeutic services, but must provide them itself. The reason is that the volume of service is too low for it to be profitable for private entrepreneurs to provide.

The market also distributes wealth unequally. The growing gap between the rich and the poor can become a source of social and political unrest. Ill health, illiteracy, lack of hygiene and sanitation, malnutrition, and crime stunt social development and may even undermine economic growth. Finally, private health care is impossibly expensive. A comparison of drug prices in Canada and the United States demonstrates the superior efficiency for the consumer of a single payer (the government), as opposed to many payers (individuals or private insurance companies). Even the rich cannot afford health care on their own, but need to share the risk of ill health and infirmity with others through insurance. Furthermore, for-profit insurance and health care delivery is based on the principle of identifying and serving the low-risk population, while the "whole point of public health insurance is to create a large, balanced risk pool."[1] For all of these reasons, *the state has come to regulate the market*.

These two functions of government—freeing business up to be more profitable and regulating it—did not come into being overnight. It took centuries for the state to evolve and create the legal and political conditions of the market to flourish, and more than a century more for it to establish a comprehensive framework to regulate it: the social or *welfare state*.²

Medicare and the other social rights are bound up with the modern social or welfare state. The fully developed welfare state differs from earlier liberal market societies in defining goods such as health care, education, income security, and housing as entitlements of all citizens and as the hallmarks of a civilized society. Such goods are no longer regarded as private responsibilities to be supplied by individual effort, charity, or punitive state efforts to discipline the workforce. As Samuel Martin puts it:

> society as a whole decrees that all its members shall be provided with an appropriate level of health care, education, cultural enjoyment and general social well-being. These shall become public, not private goods. The allocation of society's resources for the attainment of the good life shall be skimmed off the top of the national wealth in the only fair and equitable way yet devised by mankind: through a tax system imposed by a democratic government. Charity—a word with demeaning connotations—would cease to exist. Each citizen would accept humanistic service from public institutions as his or her right. Their sole obligation and responsibility would be to the state, to pay their fair share of the tax burden needed to sustain the system. The state would decide how much humanistic service and who pays. Efficient, professional, dignified, equitable, ideal.³

De-commodification and privatization

The degree to which social rights have been institutionalized can be discussed in terms of how much protection citizens have from the inequalities and risks associated with the market economy. The latter has a tendency to transform all things into commodities, i.e. objects to be bought and sold. Most people do not have the direct means of producing all the goods they need to satisfy their basic needs—shelter, food, clothing, health care, education. They must acquire these goods from others by way of exchange, by purchasing them. For most people, this means going out to work for someone else in order to generate an income, or depending on someone who receives such an income. In other words, most people must hire out their ability to work in order to secure their livelihood, or depend on someone who does. The ability to work, or labour power, is a commodity. And *in a pure market economy,* most of the things that satisfy human needs—such as health care, housing and food—are also commodities.

If such goods are commodities and the possibility of acquiring them depends simply on the ability to pay, then they can hardly be described as the objects of *universal social rights*. To become true entitlements, they must be disconnected from individuals' purchasing power and become aspects of citizenship. The basic goods that qualify us as citizens and to which we have a social right must cease to be commodities:

> As commodities in the market, workers depend for their welfare entirely on the cash nexus. The question of social rights is thus one of de-commodification, that is of granting alternative means of welfare to that of the market. De-commodification may refer either to the service rendered, or to the status of a person, but in both cases it signifies the degree to which distribution is detached from the market mechanism. This means that the mere presence of social assistance or insurance may not necessarily bring about significant de-commodification if they do not substantially emancipate individuals from market dependence.[4]

This is what medicare made possible for all Canadians. Hospital care and treatment by physicians became freely available simply on the basis of need, without regard to an individual's ability to pay. These goods ceased to be commodities and became entitlements. They were "de-commodified."

Countries such as Norway and Sweden have come closest to the model of universal social citizenship, by ensuring that the great majority of citizens directly enjoyed the benefits provided by de-commodifying programs. A single social insurance system covered everyone, and standards were established at as high a level as possible, rather than reduced to the lowest common denominator. As Esping-Andersen puts it: "This model crowds out the market and, consequently, inculcates an essentially universal solidarity behind the welfare state. All benefit, all are dependent, and all will presumably feel obliged to pay."[5] Furthermore, those countries strove to socialize the costs of care and maximize the individual's autonomy. They invested considerable resources in health, child and elder care, rather than defining them as principally the responsibility of each individual and family.

Privatization shrinks that space in which citizens are protected from the impact of the market by transforming goods such as health care into commodities. Privatization thus threatens social rights, and with them democracy. Where the social welfare state de-commodifies basic goods such as health care and education, privatization re-commodifies them.

As the antithesis of the welfare state, privatization is a broad tendency that pervades every aspect of our society today. The privatization tendencies at work in Canada's health care system are part and parcel of this general trend. It has been said that "the welfare state is about the care of dependent people. The crisis of the welfare state is at least in part (...) a crisis of the care of the dependent."[6] The cascading effect evoked by Pat Armstrong does not begin in the health care system—it would be fair to say that it has washed away social rights in many other sectors already and is only now attacking the social right to free, universal, accessible, comprehensive, portable and publicly administered health care.

How the privatization trend exploits the internal crisis of health care

This attack on health care is insidious. In part, it has taken advantage of a more general fiscal crisis of the welfare state, as we shall see in the following sections. But it has also made use of a crisis of legitimacy within health care itself.[7] For years, North America was dominated by an ideology that emphasized the *curative* function of medicine and gave all power within health care to physicians. We could call this an *aristocratic* model, in the sense that all knowledge and authority were vested in a small elite of physicians at the apex of the health care pyramid.

In recent years, this model has been challenged more and more by an ideology that stresses the prevention of illness and health promotion, that champions an integrated, holistic model of health care instead of the traditional pyramid. In this model, many other health care professions than medicine have a prominent role. Furthermore, the patient is regarded as the true centre of the process and is encouraged to be an active, knowledgeable consumer. We could call this model *democratic*.

But there is a third ideology, a *technocratic* one, pushed by administrators, bureaucrats, businessmen, and politicians, which discusses health care as an enterprise, as a business. This discourse is most concerned with investment and return on investment, with cost/benefit analysis, with risk management, with cost-containment and rationalization, with restructuring and privatization. The people who hold to this ideology have exploited dissatisfaction with traditional aristocratic medicine and the desire for change embodied in the more democratic ideology, in order to push through huge changes to our health care system—changes that are leading away from the social right to health care and towards its privatization.

In order to understand the politics and ideology of privatization, it is useful to keep these two levels in mind:
- the challenge to the welfare state and social rights as a whole, one of the main forms of which is the discourse on the debt/deficit crisis, out of which emerges a movement to cut health care spending in the name of cost-containment;
- the challenge to the traditional structure of health-care delivery in the name of patient- centered care, which can take the direction of democratization or consumerism—a political transformation of medicine or a market-driven one.

The wellspring of privatization in the Canadian state

The welfare state was heralded in the reports of the Royal Commission on Dominion-Provincial Relations (1940), the Advisory Committee on Health Insurance (1943), and the Advisory Committee on Reconstruction (1943). The construction of the welfare state took place over a thirty-year period, from the introduction of unemployment insurance in 1940 and universal family allowances in 1943, through Saskatchewan's 1946 Hospital Insurance Act, the 1957 federal Hospital Insurance and Diagnostic Services Act, the 1965 creation of the Canada and Quebec Pension Plans, the 1966 enactment of the Canada Assistance Plan and Medical Care Insurance Act, to the 1971 reform of unemployment insurance. As a result of these various measures, the Canadian state went some way towards recognizing its citizens' rights to social assistance on the basis of need, to financial assistance in raising their children, to an adequate retirement income, to social insurance against the risk of unemployment, and to medical care. After 1971, no major new social programs were introduced at the federal level, although there was some consolidation, most notably in the 1984 Canada Health Act. Unfortunately, many social programs—notably Unemployment Insurance, Old Age Security, Family Allowances, and the Canada Assistance Plan—were limited, diluted, or abolished during the 1980s and 1990s, threatening citizens' social rights.

It is a commonplace to say that the welfare state has been in crisis in all industrialized countries for two decades or more. To be sure, political scientists such as Claus Offe have argued that the welfare state is in fact intrinsically crisis-ridden.[8] However, the last decade in particular has witnessed major changes in the balance of class power and the strategies of state rule, which have seriously weakened the welfare system in the process.[9]

The welfare state developed as a way of containing social and political conflict and fueling economic growth. On the one hand, this meant appeasing popular aspirations for social change after the hardships of the Depression and especially after the Second World War. On the other hand, a key function of the welfare state was to counter the centrifugal forces within the Canadian federation—competing regions and provinces, and, underlying them, competing sectors of industry. Finally, state income redistribution programs, economic planning, and major investment projects (the St. Lawrence Seaway, highways, hospitals, universities, nuclear energy, gas and oil, hydro, etc.) contributed to, and sustained, high levels of economic growth.

This system entered a period of crisis with the stagflation of the 1970s. Economic growth rates declined while the average rate of unemployment, as well as the depth and extent of poverty, increased in each decade from the 1960s to the 1990s. The explanation of this phenomenon is a matter of considerable theoretical controversy into which it is not necessary to go here. Suffice it to say that the welfare state reached the limits of its expansion in the 1970s. In Canada, its high point came in the early 1970s, with Bryce Mackasey's extension of the unemployment insurance program and the progressive proposals contained in the social security review launched in 1973.[10]

With falling growth rates everywhere, governments came under increasing pressure from business to end re-distributive policies designed to bring about greater social equality. A notorious report by Samuel Huntington for the Trilateral Commission warned of the growing "ungovernability" of Western countries, due to the increasing politicization of social and economic life. The remedy proposed was to roll back the state, to reverse many aspects of social citizenship and decommodification, and even of political citizenship. Neo-conservatives in many countries worried that the extension of democracy posed too great a threat to economic and social stability.[11]

Inspired by these ideas, the governments of Ronald Reagan and Margaret Thatcher in the United States and Great Britain pioneered neo-liberal economic and social policies aimed at decreasing or eliminating universal social welfare programs, while increasing fiscal welfare for corporations and the wealthy. At the same time as they curbed social and economic rights, they also limited political and civil ones. The Thatcher government seriously curtailed trade union rights, restricted citizenship in the United Kingdom, and attacked the rights of gays and lesbians. Progressive alternative policy directions were demonized and destroyed.[12]

In Canada, the governments of Brian Mulroney and Jean Chrétien shifted the tax burden from richer to poorer citizens, eliminated the universality of all income security programs, capped transfers to the provinces for health care and post-secondary education before rolling them back, and set the state on the road to privatization. The result has been to increase the market dependency of working and poor Canadians, by weakening the government transfers that shored up their incomes, by leaving them more vulnerable to market forces, by compelling them to make do with reduced public services (such as health care) or purchase them privately, and by forcing them to bear a proportionately higher tax burden.

In Britain, neo-liberalism took the very explicit form of a class conflict, as the Thatcher government waged an unrelenting campaign against the power of trade unions. In Canada, the situation is more complex. While most Canadians have remained very faithful to many of the ideals of the welfare state in spite of the neo-liberal bent of their governments, and while such attitudes are especially prevalent among lower- and middle-income individuals and women [13], governments have been largely able to secure sufficient support for—or at least short-circuit mobilization against—their moves to dismantle the welfare state by invoking the urgency of tackling the debt/deficit crisis.[14] At the level of national politics, the struggle over the welfare state has principally taken the form of a *crisis of federal-provincial relations*, whereas at the provincial level in Ontario since 1995 it has taken the explicit form of a *war on the poor*.

The crisis of federal-provincial relations

Jane Jenson has suggested that Canada's welfare state, unlike those of Western Europe, was not built upon an explicit class compromise expressed in political compacts and accommodations between competing political parties.[15] Rather, it took shape in the federal-provincial struggle to shape federalism. In countries like Sweden, social-democratic parties spearheaded the introduction of the welfare state, grounding its legitimacy in the ideology of workers' citizenship rights. In Canada, by contrast, "Keynesian programs grew out of the Depression-era and wartime bureaucracies which saw the solution to the problems of the Canadian economy residing in a stronger federal government with the will to intervene in the economy in a counter-cyclical fashion."[16] In Britain, the development of the welfare state reflected the post-war power of the working class in politics. In Canada, it assumed the form of nation-building, arousing and shaping national identities, rather than class consciousness.[17] Herein lie the roots of Canadians' (especially English-Canadians') deep attachment to medicare as a part of their identity, as well as of the structural contradictions of federal-provincial relations that form an inextricable part of medicare's evolution. The Quebec-Canada dilemma has of course been very prominent in this context. Its nationalist dimensions may however obscure the extent to which it is part of a broader dynamic pitting various regional interests against each other within the Canadian state. The crisis of the welfare state in Canada has taken the form first and foremost of a crisis of federal-provincial relations.[18] Provincial demands for greater health care funding in the wake of the 2000 federal budget are just the latest manifestation of this.

Universal public health care was first introduced in Canada by the *provincial* government of Tommy Douglas in Saskatchewan. The federal government however played the leading role in establishing it across Canada. Overcoming resistance from the provinces (notably Ontario and Quebec), as well as physicians and the private insurance industry, the federal government laid the foundations of medicare in the 1957 federal Hospital Insurance and Diagnostic Services Act and the 1966 Medical Care Insurance Act.[19]

Under the constitution, the provincial governments have jurisdiction over health care and are responsible for administering and delivering health care services. The cost of health care ($ 80 billion from all sources in 1998), as of other social programs, is however beyond the financial capacity of the provinces alone. The provinces' fiscal impotence in this respect became glaringly obvious during the Great Depression. From the late 1930s on, the federal government exploited this weakness to establish a presence and active role in areas of provincial jurisdiction. While the provinces had jurisdiction over health and welfare, their fiscal capacity was limited. By virtue of the constitutional doctrine of the spending power, however, the federal government had "the right to make payments to individuals, institutions and other governments for any purpose, and to attach conditions to those payments if it wishes. More particularly, [the doctrine of the spending power] supports the right to make such payments even if the purposes involved fall fully within provincial jurisdiction, provided that they do not amount to regulation."[20] This power has been the basis for federal spending on health care. Without federal support, Canada's health care system would be fragmented and lack coherence. Canadians could not enjoy equal access to high quality, "universal, accessible, comprehensive, portable and publicly administered"[21] health care. The relative wealth of each province would dictate the quality and universality of its health care services. Even the wealthiest of provinces would be hard pressed to sustain anything approaching the existing system. Health care in Canada is thus caught—not to say trapped—in a tangled web of federal-provincial relations that are fraught with conflict and contradiction. The federal presence remains essential, both because the federal government takes a large share of available tax revenues, and because only the threat of federal money disappearing can compel provinces intent on contravening the Canada Health Act from doing so.

The federal government was able to secure provincial support for establishing public health insurance across Canada by using its spending power to share the costs of the system with the provinces. By the late 1970s, however, as the cost of medicare constantly increased, Ottawa pulled out of cost-sharing. Under the existing open-ended shared-cost formula, the federal government was faced with ballooning, unpredictable spending requirements, a problem not fully solved by changes to the funding formula introduced in the early 1970s. Provincial governments, for their part, considered that the cost-sharing arrangements allowed the federal government to interfere too much in areas of provincial responsibility, and at the same time did not guarantee a sufficiently stable and predictable funding base. For these reasons, both levels of government saw a shift to federal block grants as advantageous. The result was the *Federal-Provincial Fiscal Arrangements and Federal Post-Secondary Education and Health Contributions Act, 1977*[22], commonly known as Established Programs Financing, or EPF.

With the advent of Established Programs Financing, a single funding formula covered three of the major cost-sharing programs (hospital insurance, medicare, and post-secondary education). Cost-sharing was replaced by block funding comprised of transferred federal taxation powers ("tax room") and cash payments, and subjected to levelling and transitional adjustments.

The federal government first reduced personal and corporate taxes.[23] This allowed the provinces to raise their taxes by an equivalent amount without causing taxpayers to pay more overall. Furthermore, because the transfer of tax points alone did not enable less prosperous provinces to generate the revenue they needed, Ottawa granted them additional equalization payments.

Each province then received cash on top of the transferred tax points. The EPF transfer was to grow each year according to a formula based on the growth of Gross National Product (GNP) and provincial population.[24] Each province received an amount equal to the national per capita federal government contribution multiplied by that province's population. Hospital insurance and medicare were allocated 71.25% of the transfer, while the remaining 28.75% were to be spent on post-secondary education. The national per capita contribution was based on the federal per capita contribution in the first year of the arrangement (1975-76), indexed every year to the moving average over three years of the growth in the Gross National Product per capita.

EPF transfers began to be cut back almost from the start, beginning in the early 1980s with the Trudeau government's 6 & 5 anti-inflation program, the Mulroney government's Bill C-96 in 1986, which decreased the EPF GNP escalator to the rate of growth of GNP minus 2%, the 1990 federal budget, which froze the EPF per capita cash transfer to the provinces for two years, and the 1991 federal budget, which extended the freeze on EPF cash transfers until 1995.

The five-year (1990-1995) freeze imposed by the 1990 and 1991 changes entailed huge losses of revenue for the provinces. In the name of trimming the deficit, the Mulroney government, "through its unilateral changes to EPF funding, deliberately added $41 billion to provincial debts and deficits for the 1986-1995 period."[25] The effects of all of these cuts were cumulative. Changes made to EPF transfers in the early 1980s still reverberated a decade later. Beyond the fiscal consequences of offloading the debt on the provinces, the freeze on EPF cash transfers and subsequent cuts jeopardized national standards in health care. Extrapolating from current trends in the early 1990s, the National Council of Welfare and other analysts predicted the end of the EPF cash transfer by the year 2000.[26] Thereafter, they would consist only of "tax room"; there would be no cash component left. Given the uneven wealth of the various provinces, a given portion of tax room means an unequal amount of tax raised per capita in each province. The cash outlay was meant to ensure that each province got the same per capita amount. If health care and post-secondary education were ever to be funded "exclusively by taxes raised by provincial and territorial governments," the National Union of Public and General Employees warned, "national standards will be a thing of the past, and provincial programs will be a direct function of the ability of individual provinces to raise enough money from their own residents from taxation, user fees, and other means."[27]

Meanwhile, transfers for social assistance and social services under the Canada Assistance Plan (CAP) were supposed to be cost-shared on a 50:50 basis. But in 1991, the Mulroney government imposed its notorious "cap on CAP," limiting increases in the CAP transfer to the three wealthiest provinces, Ontario, Alberta and British Columbia, to a maximum of 5 percent a year. By 1994, the federal contribution to Ontario under the Canada Assistance Plan was down to 29 percent of provincial expenditures on social assistance and social services covered by CAP. As a result, while Quebec, for example, was receiving $3,300 from Ottawa for every social assistance recipient, Ontario was getting only $1,800.[28] In the context of the deep recession and the tens of thousands of layoffs following the signing of the Canada-U.S. Free Trade Agreement, these cuts had a devastating impact on provincial finances.

The 1995 federal budget announced the fusion of EPF with the Canada Assistance Plan in a new block fund, to be called the Canada Social Transfer (soon renamed Canada Health and Social Transfer, or CHST). In addition to eliminating CAP's cost-sharing for social assistance and social services, the federal government cut the total cash transfer to the provinces by a third, or about $6 billion out of $18 billion. The combination of EPF and CAP shored up the cash component of the block fund, putting off the date of its ultimate demise—but only at the cost of leaving the provinces with much less money and pitting health care and post-secondary education against social assistance. Nevertheless, under the CHST too the cash component was scheduled to disappear. According to statistical analysis by Matt Sanger, the federal CHST cash transfer to Ontario, for example, would have fallen from $6.3 billion in 1994/1995 to $96 million in 2003/2004, and nothing at all the following year.[29] During the 1997 federal election campaign, the Liberal Party promised to maintain the cash component at $12.5 billion. The 1998, 1999 and 2000 post-deficit federal budgets increased this amount for the years up to 2004. The cash transfer to all the provinces was scheduled to reach $15.5 billion that year—still well short of the more than $18 billion in cash transferred to them in 1995.[30] However, the September 2000 health-care agreement between the First Ministers promises to restore the cash transfer to $18.3 billion in 2001-2002, and $21 billion in 2005-2006. Still, federal cuts will have had a harsh impact on the provinces.

Federal cash transfers to Ontario under EPF dropped after 1993-1994, even though the tax component of the transfer continued to increase. The truly crushing blow came in the wake of the 1995 federal budget. In 1995-1996, the combined EPF/CAP cash entitlement was $6.2 billion. In 1996-1997, it fell to $4.7 billion, and a year later to $3.8 billion. The extent of the cutbacks is even more blatant when measured in constant dollars and per capita. In 2000 dollars, the combined CAP/EPF cash

Table 1
Federal transfers to Ontario under EPF/CAP and CHST, 1994-2000
(constant 2000 $)

	1994-1995	1995-1996	1996-1997	1997-1998	1998-1999	1999-2000
Health care price index, Ontario (2000=100)	91.2	92.5	93.9	95.6	98.9	100.0
Population of Ontario (thousands)	10,828	10,965	11,101	11,260	11,412	11,549
Total EPF-CAP/CHST transfer (millions)	11,553	11,610	10,278	9,744	9,825	10,968
EPF-CAP/CHST tax transfer (millions)	4,604	4,892	5,180	5,678	5,927	6,129
EPF-CAP/CHST cash transfer (millions)	6,948	6,719	5,098	4,066	3,898	4,840
Total EPF-CAP/CHST per capita transfer	1,067	1,059	926	865	861	950
EPF-CAP/CHST per capita tax transfer	425	446	467	504	519	531
EPF-CAP/CHST per capita cash transfer	642	613	459	361	342	419

Sources: Federal and Provincial Relations Division, Department of Finance, Canada, February 2000; Statistics Canada, CANSIM Matrix P106085 (inflation projected at 3% in 2000-2001); Canadian Institute for Health Information (population growth projected at 1.298% 2000-2001 forward); Bill Murnighan, "Health Care Spending in Ontario," Ontario Alternative Budget Working Group, Paper No. 8, April 2000.

transfer to Ontario was $6.9 billion in 1994-1995; in 1998-1999, it had dropped to $3.9 billion, a cumulative loss of some $8 billion over four years. In per capita terms, it had plummeted from $642 to $342. The 2002-2006 increase in the CHST cash transfer promised by the federal government in September 2000 will amount to about $8 billion for Ontario. It will thus at best restore what was taken away between 1995 and 1999. Ontario will have lost years' worth of potential investments in health care as a result of the federal government's disastrous cuts of the mid-1990s (see Table 1).

The Harris government, and the Rae government before it, have constantly complained about federal cutbacks. There is indeed little doubt that the latter have hit Ontario hard. On the other hand, provincial outrage over transfer-payment reductions since 1995 has to be placed in the context of the provincial government's policy of diminishing its own fiscal capacity by reducing income taxes substantially—a reduction, moreover, that has disproportionately benefited wealthier Ontarians: "Fifty-seven percent of the benefit goes to the highest-income 20 percent of households; only 1 percent of the benefit goes to the lowest-income 20 percent of households. The middle 50 percent of households, ranked by income, receive only 35 percent of the gain from the tax cut."[31] The province could have chosen not to give wealthy citizens a hefty income-tax break, and instead collected the taxes and spent them on health care.

After the introduction of EPF in 1977, the federal government faced the political conundrum that it was transferring increasing amounts of money to the provinces for health care and post- secondary education, without any way of controlling how the provinces spent it, indeed without any guarantee that they would even spend it in those areas rather than on tax cuts, for example, and without getting any real credit from the general public. In the case of health care, this changed somewhat after the 1984 passage of the Canada Health Act which put a stop to the practice of extra-billing by physicians. In addition to enshrining national standards for health care in law, the Canada Health Act made it much more difficult for the provinces to shift health care costs to private payers. It enabled the federal government to present itself as the great defender of Canada's most cherished social program against the provinces.

However, many would argue that *both* levels of government today are pursuing the same underlying social agenda, the re-commodification of the de-commodified sectors of health care and post-secondary education. They are both actively promoting the greater market dependency of working people and the poor by cutting back on income-security programs such as unemployment insurance and social assistance, and favouring other programs (such as the national child benefit) which are designed as "incentives to work." This "re-commodification" agenda is manifest in the promotion of "public-private partnerships" and the commercialization of public services. Yet, given very high levels of public support for medicare, both levels of government must pay lip service to the Canada Health Act and public health care. At stake in their struggle

The war on the poor

The Harris government was first elected in June 1995 on a platform it called the "Common Sense Revolution."[32] Common sense, as everyone knows, is as old as the hills, the compendium of experience, tradition and prejudice. It is inherently bound to the way things are or appear to be in the light of popular wisdom or everyday forms of reasoning. The idea of revolution by contrast suggests something overwhelming, all-encompassing and new. In fact, the Common Sense Revolution was neither revolutionary, in the sense of involving radical innovation, nor commonsensical—rather, it echoed the ideas and policies of Anglo-American conservatives since the 1970s. It consisted of a potent neo-conservative brew of neo-liberal economics and "authoritarian populist" social policy. Neo-liberal economics rejects the welfare state and advocates privatization, because it believes that the market is the most efficient mechanism for allocating resources in society. Authoritarian populism for its part attacks the welfare state as encouraging immoral, deviant and criminal behaviour that undermines the central social institutions of work, family and state.[33]

Neo-liberal market philosophy holds that a strictly capitalist society provides greater individual freedom than any other form of social order: it frees individuals from the tyranny of the state and dependence on others, subjects them all equally to the forces of the market, and allows them to succeed or fail on the basis of their own abilities, initiative, risk-taking and hard work. In this scenario there needs to be a strong state to ensure that the rules of the marketplace and the sanctity of private property are respected by all. Beyond this, however, the state must not interfere with the workings of the market. All forms of government regulation of the economy, whether of financial markets through regulations on banks or of labour markets through minimum wage legislation, laws guaranteeing trade union rights, unemployment insurance, etc. are regarded by neo-conservatives with considerable reservations, if not outright suspicion.

While most believers in the neo-liberal market philosophy would accept the need for some support for the destitute, the sick and the elderly, this is to be kept to a minimum so as to interfere as little as possible with market outcomes. In the words of Mike Harris, borrowing from Bill Clinton during the 1995 general election campaign, the aim of welfare should be to give people "a hand up, not a hand-out." It follows from these ideas that the welfare state with its large public sector must be unproductive and parasitical, leeching wealth away from those sectors that create it (i.e. business) and giving it to those that do not (i.e. the poor, public servants).

This is the philosophy behind the policies introduced by the Harris government:
- the large income tax cuts, which have been compensated for by reductions in public services, by the introduction of new or increased user charges, and by the downloading of a number of provincial responsibilities to other levels of government;
- the massive attack on trade union rights and employment standards (Bills 7 and 136);
- drastic restriction of access to social assistance, huge cuts to benefits, and stringent pay-back conditions imposed on social assistance recipients, as well as recipients of day-care subsidies;
- the centralization of bureaucratic and political control over the public sector and broader public sector;
- the weakening of local democracy at the municipal, school board, and district health council levels.

"Steering, not rowing"? Applying private-sector management ideology to the public sector

The PC Party of Ontario's 1995 election campaign platform, the *Common Sense Revolution*, declared:
> It's time for us to take a fresh look at government. To re-invent the way it works, to make it work for people. (...) we are governed by a system that was designed to meet the needs of the 1950s, not the challenges of the 1990s or beyond.[34]

It promised to transform public administration in Ontario by demanding "that government [do] business *like* a business, [i.e.] in an efficient and productive manner that focuses on results and puts the customer first." To this end, the PC Party promised to reduce the cost of public administration by cutting "fat" and "non-priority government spending"[35], doing away with "red tape" and "over-regulation," reducing taxes, setting performance standards for public services, encouraging departments to save money," selling off government assets, doing "better with less," and looking "at creative ideas for increasing the private sector's role.[36] This program also gave away the cost of these policies: 13,000 public servants were to be laid off.

The 1995 Ontario Throne Speech announced that the government would review all of its activities and shed all those that would best be left to others, such as individuals, communities or the private sector—and the government would consequently shed all the people who had been doing that work. It would also identify the best delivery agents and strategies for the services it still intended to provide. Such strategies could include public-private partnerships, licensing and franchising, purchasing services from the private sector, as well as allowing outside agencies to compete with government ones.

In February 1996, the Ontario Management Board approved an alternative-service-delivery framework that established "the guiding principles, range of service delivery options and selection criteria to help ministries choose the most appropriate delivery option for a particular program."[37] Under this framework, each ministry was to prepare an annual business plan, outline its restructuring proposals, and recommend measures to redesign, eliminate, or deliver programs more efficiently using alternative delivery methods. Ministries were also provided with guidelines for reviewing and redesigning programs, as well as selecting alternative service delivery options.[38]

On reviewing each program, ministries were to decide either to continue offering services if they were affordable, to sell them off if they no longer served the public interest, or to abolish them outright should their mandate no longer be "in line with government policy." The government was to continue providing a service itself "only if this [were] the best way of serving the public interest"; the reasons for doing so would have to be "conclusive." Service delivery models would be based on "a solid analysis of cost-effectiveness, ensuring good customer service and the best possible return on tax dollars." If the government were to offer the service itself, it would "[manage] the delivery of these services like a business." The government would remain accountable to the public *for the results*; it would be considered legitimate for the private-sector to make profits from delivering public services, provided "the government [achieved] its policy objectives."[39] A number of government activities were deemed unsuitable for privatization:

Activities that require daily directives and policy interpretation do not lend themselves readily to new modes of service delivery. Here are some examples:
I. policy analysis and development; development of new programs and changes to programs; development of legislative proposals;
II. intergovernmental relations;

III. proposed regulations; formulation of standards;

IV. programs with a large equity and justice component.⁴⁰

The plan, then, was first to establish a clear demarcation line between legislative and policy-related matters on the one hand, and the delivery of services on the other; secondly to distinguish between the ends and the means of service delivery (government would be accountable for the *results*, not the ways of achieving them); and thirdly, to treat service delivery strictly in market terms (it would be managed like a business, be based on a solid analysis of cost-effectiveness, yield a good return on investment, and ensure customer satisfaction).

In keeping with this, each ministry is required to publish annual "business plans"; the Ministry of Health's business plans refer to its major program areas, such as hospitals, physician care, drugs and devices, etc., as "core businesses." Since 1998-1999, the core businesses in the Ministry of Health are defined as community services, professional services, institutional services, and policy and planning. These categories represent the functions respectively of health promotion, prevention, and home care; care by health professionals, including physicians of course, but also nurse practitioners, midwives, and various kinds of therapists represented by Ontario's twenty-two colleges of health professionals; care in hospitals and long-term-care facilities; and decision-making and outcome-measurement.

The alternative-service-delivery options considered included: privatization (defined as "[selling] the asset or its controlling interest in a service to a private sector business"); franchises and licencing; public-private partnerships; buying outside services; transfer of responsibilities (to municipalities, transfer-payment agencies, or grant-receiving non-profit organizations); government- controlled agencies; or direct delivery by the goverment.⁴¹

These ideas were scarcely original. On the contrary, they were extremely fashionable in the mid-1990s. They repeated what many other governments were saying throughout North America and the English-speaking world, where public administration has been restructured in the name of new frameworks of accountability based on measurement of outcomes, performance indicators, etc.⁴² For example, the federal government's Program Review process initiated by Marcel Massé in 1994 is based on strikingly similar guidelines.⁴³ These ideas are encapsulated in the slogan of *entrepreneurial government* expressed in David Osborne and Ted Gaebler's best-selling book, *Reinventing Government*:

> Most entrepreneurial governments promote *competition* between service providers. They *empower* citizens by pushing con-

trol out of the bureaucracy, into the community. They measure the performance of their agencies, focussing not on inputs but on *outcomes*. They are driven by their goals—their *missions*—not by their rules and regulations. They redefine their clients as *customers* and offer them choices—between schools, between training programs, between housing options. They *prevent* problems before they emerge, rather than simply offering services afterward. They put their energies into *earning* money, not simply spending it. They *decentralize* authority, embracing participatory management. They prefer *market* mechanisms to bureaucratic mechanisms. And they focus not simply on providing public services, but on *catalysing* all sectors—public, private, and voluntary—into action to solve their community's problems.[44]

Despite the rhetorical emphasis on participation, such reforms do not lean in the direction of genuine democratization, but rather toward the market. Their core values are not social justice and citizenship, but efficiency, productivity and consumerism. Paul Thomas's comments highlight the themes shared by the Harris, Chrétien and Clinton governments[45]:

Reinventing government consists of cutting back to basics, removing red tape, putting customers first, making governments more business-like and revenue dependent, and searching for continuous improvement in programs. The Chrétien government's slogan for the new approach is "smarter and more affordable government," which bears a strong resemblance to the Clinton administration's motto of creating a government that "works better and costs less."[46]

It is evident that to claim that the Harris government's outlook was derivative, rather than original, is not to say that it could not have made other choices or that it does not bear the full responsibility for the consequences of those choices. It is rather to understand that the Harris government's agenda in many ways coincides with a more general trend, the transition from a welfare state focussed on ideals of social citizenship and providing some measure of *de-commodification*, to a neo-liberal state focussed on market value and pursuing the goal of *re-commodification*. Situating the Ontario government's ideology and policies in that broader context enables us to understand them not as the whims of a few politicians, but as deeper political trends driven by the shifting balance of forces between classes and regions in Canadian society.

The Harris government's agenda and the neo-liberal managerial ideology

The Harris government's agenda incorporates many of the values associated with the shift from the "fordist" mass production of services to "post-fordism."[47] Robin Murray and others have suggested that the postwar welfare state in Canada and elsewhere "was organized on principles and institutions similar to those of mass production"; they refer to it as a "fordist" state characterized by: (1) "mass production of standardized services"; (2) "economies of scale" (bigger schools, hospitals); (3) "administration through multi-divisional forms of organization, adopted from the managerial models of large private companies"; (4) application of the "principles of time economy (...) to the actual delivery of the service, processing the users to suit the time and balance-sheet requirements of the producer." Examples include increasing the number of "induced births in maternity care in order to minimize deliveries on weekends." Another example is the "use of queues and waiting time to manage fluctuations in demand on capacity." The result was "a trend towards the 'deskilling' of users in particular state services, such as health."[48] According to George Torrance, the general pattern for health care in Western welfare states consisted of:

> a heavy emphasis on curative medicine as enshrined in private practice and acute-treatment hospitals and little attention to the socio-economic sources of illness, prevention, public health, or rehabilitation; a complex and expensive medical technology; the growth of specialization at the expense of primary care; a rigid division of labour that discouraged the reallocation of roles; the creation of new sources of corporate profits and professional wealth from state-subsidized care; and the intrusion of the medical industry into a range of problems that were formerly considered outside its competence.[49]

The last two decades have witnessed a crisis of the fordist model. But instead of following the path of democratic participation and administration, the powers that be opted for market strategies. These entailed significant transformations in the organization of production, a shift from the mass production of standardized goods and services in large vertically integrated factories and organizations to diversified production of more specialized goods and services in more streamlined, horizontally integrated, units of production.

This has been reflected in the public sector as well, as ministries, agencies and other institutions have been "re-engineered" along the principles of new public management theories. Like their private sector counterparts, many public institutions have redefined their mandates, contracted out and commercialized many of their activities, laid off part of their workforce, and sought to manage their operations on market-like principles. An example of such a change is the move to shift patient care away from general hospitals—conceived from a management perspective as large vertically integrated "health factories"[50] producing a comprehensive array of services—towards a variety of smaller-scale services, such as home care, chronic care and long-term care, in which labour costs are lower. Sociologists have referred to the new model of private and public sector production and management as "post-fordism."[51]

The May 1996 Ontario Ministry of Health *Business Plan* presents a vision and mission that echo many of these themes. It promised a seamless, *integrated, patient-centred* health care system, in which resources would be equitably distributed throughout the province. It announced that the government would cease to be a "passive payer and service provider," and would instead become an "active manager that integrates the components of the system, encourages effective partnerships and strategically manages information." To this end, the government would "explore divesting direct services" by transferring them to the non-profit or private sectors. It would measure the system's performance on the basis of the results achieved.[52] The statement appeared to subscribe to a number of Osborne and Gaebler's ten principles of entrepreneurial government: steering rather than rowing (i.e. setting policy instead of delivering services directly); funding outcomes, not inputs; leveraging change through the market; injecting competition into service delivery; meeting the needs of the customer, not the bureaucracy.[53] In this scenario, patients become customers, service delivery is contracted out to the agency that can provide it most cheaply; service is defined in terms of a restricted number of measurable goals or "outputs." In Chapters 2 and, especially, 3, we shall see what such "alternative service delivery" has really meant in practice in Ontario's health care system.

In 1996, under Bill 26, the Harris government established the Health Services Restructuring Commission (HSRC), "a stand-alone corporation, with a four-year mandate, operating at arm's length from the Government of Ontario." The Commission was granted "the authority to restructure hospitals in Ontario" and to make "recommendations to the Minister of Health on restructuring other elements of the health services system." The HSRC was given a four-year mandate until March 1999. One of the HSRC's first acts was to propose a general vision of the future of health care in Ontario. In a nutshell, it proposed a fully integrated system centred no longer on hospitals, but on rostered populations, who would gain access to primary, community, ambulatory, specialist, hospital, and long-term care from a single access point. The provincial government would set the overall goals of the health system through legislation, policy, regulation, standards. It would also be responsible for funding the system on a capitation basis. "Responsibility and accountability for operational decision-making, program/service delivery, and performance outcomes [would] rest with regionally-oriented integrated health systems (IHSs) and regional integrated academic health systems (IAHSs)." These regional bodies would create formal networks of hospitals, physicians and other providers. They would (1) "serve the health needs of a geographic or, in large municipalities with a number of IHSs, faith-based, ethnic, or other rostered population (size: 100,000 to 500,000)," (2) "manage a fixed, predetermined pool of funds to provide a comprehensive package of services to a defined, registered population (i.e. capitation funding)," (3) "provide or purchase defined services on behalf of the people registered," (4) "assume responsibility for providing defined services in return for payment (i.e. provide a full range of primary and secondary services, long-term, community, and facility-based care and palliative care)." The vision statement concluded with a list of policy issues the HSRC intended to pursue. These included integrated delivery, capitation, rostering, structured competition among integrated delivery systems, health care report cards, and public-private partnerships.[54]

Ideological overlaps and ambiguities: What does integration really mean?

State regulation of social life has both positive and negative dimensions. It can signify protecting citizens from the arbitrariness and violence of oppressive personal relationships—protection of children from parental violence and neglect is an obvious example. At the same time it may simply replace unchecked personal domination by alienating, impersonal bureaucratic rule. The collective mobilization which led to the consolidation of the welfare state aimed for universally accessible, free education and health services. However, government intervention too often produced services in which "client" populations were dependent on the state, and in which a hierarchical division of labour among the service-providers led to domination of knowledge holders and planners over de-skilled executors.[55]

The state appropriates the various forms of knowledge related to education, health, housing, and so on, which had up till then either been widely distributed among the population, or had been controlled by relatively unregulated professional bodies. These various bodies of knowledge then get crystallized in more and more specialized professional corporations in the same process that transforms public into state services. In this way, a veritable cultural dispossession of user populations occurs, as the latter find themselves separated from monopolized forms of knowledge, excluded from any ability to undertake certain forms of services, and by that token subjected to state institutions.[56]

The result of this process is increasing dependency of those who use public services on experts and state bureaucracies, even within the de-commodified spheres that are supposed to enhance social citizenship. Health care is of course a prime example of this, but so are education and welfare. More and more social situations become technical problems to be resolved administratively by experts, instead of political issues to be resolved through a democratic process by service users and providers. The increasing prevalence among government agencies of management strategies imported from private business has reinforced this tendency, by increasing the dispossession not just of users with respect to providers, but also of workers with respect to managers within government bureaucracies.

The medical profession in Canada had consolidated itself and achieved a hegemonic position within health care before the rise of the welfare state. And while physicians' associations waged a losing battle against the introduction of medicare, they were successful in retaining most of their power in the system. As Torrance puts it,

> they retained almost total control over the content of their work, and in many cases control as well over the way health care was organized. (...) fee-for-service was still a prevalent form of payment. Medical control over key institutions like hospitals and paramedical occupations went unchallenged. Thus the introduction of state health insurance or health services tended to freeze the patterns of organization that existed at the time of implementation.[57]

The fordist model may have offered a minimum of public services to all citizens, but it tended to do so in a bureaucratic fashion, in which the citizens receiving the services had little say in how their needs were defined or would be addressed.[58] In tandem with the shift from fordism to post-fordism, the curative model of health care has been called into question and there has been greater (at least rhetorical) emphasis on the socio-economic determinants of health. Critics of medicine pointed out that the latter had developed an exclusively bio-medical pathology and lacked a socio-economic perspective on the causes of disease. Instead of pumping resources into a system designed to cure people once they become sick, and which treats them as the passive recipients of medical wizardry, this line of thinking stresses both the need to prevent illness in the first place and to empower citizens to deal with disease themselves. This is not new—19th-century social reformers had already linked poverty and insalubrious housing to the incidence of morbidity. Dr. Norman Bethune, a Canadian pioneer in the treatment of tuberculosis, had already campaigned in the 1930s for the eradication of the social causes of the disease.[59] Such ideas regained currency in the 1970s and after, thanks to new research. Popular movements to set up community health centres or for the official recognition of midwifery are reactions to this phenomenon.[60]

Governments have not ignored this shift. For example, the federal government's 1974 report, *A New Perspective on the Health of Canadians*, proposed "an agenda to promote the health of the Canadian population." The report called for emphasis to be placed on health, rather than health care, arguing that the latter is only one of many factors that influence health—including human biology, lifestyle, and the social and physical environments—and that they must all be addressed in order to optimize population health. The report has been criticized for focusing too narrowly on individual lifestyle choices and not enough on broader social and economic determinants.

> While the statement acknowledges that social environment can affect health, the emphasis was very much on the "choices" individuals make to engage in unhealthy behaviour. According to the Report, "personal decisions and habits that are bad from a health point of view create self-imposed risks. When those risks result in illness or death, the victim's lifestyle can be said to have contributed to, or caused, his own illness or death." There was no acknowledgement that social and economic circumstances determine the kind of "choices" individuals can make.[61]

By spreading and legitimizing the view that individuals are the authors of their own good or bad health, such ideas could even be used to legitimize cuts to public health care. By contrast, a number of important recent studies and campaigns have specifically called attention to the need to transform prevailing social and economic conditions in order to enhance public health.[62] In fact, such is the tenor of most provincial governments' reviews of their health care systems.[63]

The fordist model of health care centred on acute-care hospitals has thus been regarded as too expensive and as being the wrong model for promoting a healthier population. Critics have argued for a shift towards cheaper and more effective strategies, such as preventative medicine, community care, integrated health and social services, the use of midwives and nurse practitioners, and so on.

As I noted at the beginning of this chapter, there are three major ideologies in Anglo-American health care: a traditional ideology that emphasizes the curative activities of individual physicians; a recent ideology of health promotion and prevention; and a discourse of cost-containment and rationalization. Most progressive health critics appear to subscribe to the vision of an integrated, patient-centred health care system based on the values of wellness and prevention, fusing health and social services, moving care where appropriate out of hospitals and into the community and the home. The progressive critics of course prefer public and non-profit financing and delivery, and reject both private, for-profit service agencies and market-style structures and incentives.

However, this has given rise to a strange ambiguity, for many of these services, such as home care or midwifery, are not included in the Canada Health Act as "insured health services,"[64] and only incompletely covered by public health insurance. As Pat Armstrong has argued, an apparently progressive discourse of community care, which borrows a great deal from feminist critiques of health care, may serve here as "the legitimation for the privatization process"[65]:

> Much of the language and evidence used to justify reform is taken from the most progressive, and often feminist, critics of the health care system. (...) A variety of provincially-funded reports claim, for example, that physicians over-prescribe and over-treat, that fee-for-service encourages expenditures, and that many tests are inappropriately ordered. Some advocate more responsibility for nurse-practitioners and more culturally-sensitive care.[66]

Lip-service is paid to the progressive critiques of health care, but the market is then invoked as the solution, especially in the context of rhetoric about health care no longer being affordable in a time of fiscal crisis.

Both public education and health care have been dominated by entrenched bureaucracies and a closed elite holding a monopoly of knowledge. Citizens are increasingly speaking up in both sectors and demanding a say. But where progressive critics of these systems see the *democratization* of knowledge and administration as the answer, neo-liberals propose *market solutions*. They claim that education and health care are commodities, students and patients are customers, and that the institutions that provide them ought to operate like commercial enterprises. But as any parent or hospital patient can attest, there is a world of difference between a commercial transaction and the patient-physician or patient-nurse relationship.

There is a further important dimension to this. Colleen Fuller points out that full integration of the health care system would require the creation of centralized management systems able to handle and co-ordinate huge quantities of information and resources:

> A fully integrated delivery system, or IDS, combines physician, acute care, post-acute care, outpatient services, home care, prevention, and wellness services under a single management and financial entity. IDS depends heavily on centralized planning and information systems, which are needed to track patients through the network and provide that "seamless continuum" of care. While such highly integrated networks have not been fully established in Canada, they are emerging as the pressure to pool resources and tap new streams of revenue pushes Canadian hospitals into alliances with one another and with the corporate sector.[67]

In fact, there are moves in this direction in Ontario—one need only look at the studies produced by and for the Ontario Hospital Association on ways of building networks of hospitals, indeed, of transforming hospitals into geographically and institutionally diverse networks serving a variety of populations across the full spectrum of acute care and beyond.[68]

Robin Murray points out that according to today's management theory, "the key to corporate competitiveness (...) is how to restructure—and it is a question equally for the public sector. Until now, the skills of restructuring have been confined to capitalist management." Restructuring means reorganizing the labour process within the firm in the context of a redefinition of the firm's goals and overall strategy. As Murray points out, "any one firm is part of a much wider circuit of capital. There will usually be a dominant point in that circuit, which, if monopolized, will allow the controllers to syphon off excess profits from the circuit as a whole. These are the commanding heights of a sector."[69] The corporations that command those heights thus may have no interest in assuming ownership of hospitals or entire health networks. They need only control "the supply of primary product technology, of advanced management systems, and of international marketing."[70] Here the public and quasi-public sectors operate as markets for private corporations that supply them with technology, information management systems, management services, pharmaceutical products, medical supplies, and equipment.

Conclusion

This chapter has highlighted the politics and ideology of privatization. I have argued that privatization is not one or several *isolated or separate events*, but rather a *process* which has a cascading motion. I started from the premise that privatization is the antithesis of the welfare state. The latter *de-commodifies* health care: it takes it out of the market where individuals have to purchase it themselves, and provides it to them at no direct cost, as a social right. As a component of the welfare state, medicare creates a protected space in which citizens are sheltered from market forces.

Privatization dismantles these sheltered places and exposes citizens once again to the play of the market. It is as though the government were to sell off all the national parks to private businesses which then turned them into theme parks, private game preserves, logging zones, and shopping centres.

I then argued that the privatization cascade begins with the federal government. I discussed the latter's turn to neo-liberalism and the way this affected health care by the changes it caused in federal-provincial relations. Following from that, I sketched the neo-conservative outlook of the PC Party in Ontario and then analyzed its vision of how government (and health care in particular) should operate. I concluded with some comments on how the notion of integrated health care delivery sits at the intersection of competing ideologies of health care. The result of this, as Pat Armstrong and Colleen Fuller have argued, is an ideological ambiguity that can provide a cover for political and economic forces pushing a privatization agenda.

Chapter 2
"Cascading Privatization":
2. The Impact on Health Care Services

"We've had a vision [of health care in the Ontario government]; it's been to cut spending. (...) We're into cost-shifting and getting costs off the public books, not cost saving. Less than 70 percent of total health spending is now public and the areas where prices are rising are the private ones."[1]

Introduction

The Harris government did not wait to articulate its vision of alternative service delivery before plunging ahead and setting Ontario's health care system on the road to further privatization. The first thing it did was to introduce new user charges and significantly to cut its spending on health care (its frequent claims to have increased health care spending notwithstanding), as well as to enact legislation to give itself sweeping powers to close, amalgamate and restructure hospitals and primary care, the core services insured by medicare.

Scarcely a month after being elected, the Conservative government announced an anti-deficit program consisting of $1.9 billion in immediate spending cuts, including a $132 million reduction in health spending for 1995-1996.[2] But the cuts did not end there. The November 1995 *Fiscal and Economic Statement* stated the government's intention to restructure the financing and delivery of health services.[3] Apart from some minor investments in a few areas and the expression of some general policies (e.g., improving health services in Northern Ontario), the gist of the announcement for health care was a $1,307,000,000 cut in hospital budgets for 1996-1999 (the third year of cuts was not carried out), and the introduction of user charges for the Ontario Drug Benefit plan and patients in hospitals waiting for beds in nursing homes.

This accelerated the ongoing privatization process in hospitals. Many had long since adopted their own models of alternative service delivery and resorted to restructuring, re-engineering, outsourcing, public-private partnerships and the like. Shortened lengths of stay in hospitals, and the growing practice of treating people on an out-patient basis instead of as in-patients, shifted more and more patients from the fully insured sector of the hospital to long-term community care (nursing homes and home care), where public health coverage has stricter limits (e.g., with respect to the number of hours of nursing care to which a person is entitled, or to the availability of medical supplies and equipment). The overall impact of early restructuring and spending cuts was to create a climate of crisis—a potentially propitious situation in which to effect profound changes. This was the time when the Minister of Education, John Snobelen, was revealed to have told his top officials that the government needed to create an atmosphere of crisis in the education system in order to justify wide-ranging reforms.

This chapter provides an overview of restructuring and privatization in various sectors of the health care system, beginning with the overall financial picture, followed by sections on legislative changes, hospitals, long-term care, ambulance services, public health, user charges, and primary care. The same scenario is repeated from sector to sector: reduced spending, pressure to substitute less skilled for more skilled workers, moves to contract out services or enter into public-private partnerships.

Cutting health care expenditures

When the Progressive Conservative Party of Mike Harris won the 1995 Ontario election, the provincial deficit was $10 billion out of a total budget of $56 billion[4]—a situation brought on largely by the deepest recession in sixty years, combined with huge cuts in transfer payments received from the federal government for health care, post-secondary education, social assistance and social services. Yet, the Harris government promised to balance the budget *and* cut taxes by an average of 30 percent. This suggested that huge spending cuts were on the way. Nonetheless, the government promised to improve health care without reducing public funding or increasing private costs. The PC Party's election platform, *The Common Sense Revolution*, stated unequivocally: "We will not cut health care spending. It's far too important... Under this plan, health care spending will be guaranteed." Claiming that money could be saved by "rooting out waste, abuse, health-card fraud, mismanagement and duplication, " the Conservatives promised to reinvest all savings in direct care, putting "an end to rationing and waiting lists."[5] Although the Conservative government began its mandate with hundreds of millions of dollars of health care spending cuts, it has since made many new spending announcements. In the spring of 2000, it has launched a major television advertising campaign to tell the public that it has greatly increased health care expenditures, while the federal government has cut back. As we saw in Chapter 1, the latter is true. But what of the former? Has the Ontario government significantly increased health care spending?

Notwithstanding the Ontario government's spring 2000 ideological offensive to prove that it has boosted health care spending, the record shows that health care, like other sectors, has fared poorly under the Conservative government. Table 2 shows total operating expenditures on health care declining in constant dollars for four straight years, from 1994-1995 to 1997-1998. Health care spending did not get back to 1993-1994 levels until 1998-1999.

Per capita health expenditures by the province declined from 1995 to 2000. They fell from an average of $1,790 in 1995 to $1,682 in 1998. In 1999-2000, they will have risen to $1,722, still short of their 1995 level. In fact, the cumulative loss to Ontario's health care system since 1995 from the cuts made by the provincial government will amount to nearly $3 billion in 2001.

Between 1985 and 1991, private sector health expenditures in Ontario diminished sharply in comparison with provincial government ones (from a ratio of 29 percent private to 71 percent public in 1985, to one of 26 percent private to 74 percent public in 1991). However, from 1992 on, private health care spending began to gain ground on provincial government health care expenditures (from a ratio of 27 percent private to 73 percent public in 1992, to one of 29 percent private to 71

Table 2
Provincial government expenditures on health care, Ontario, 1994-2001

Year	Provincial government expenditures on health care* (current $ millions)	Health care price index, Ontario (2000=100)	Provincial government expenditures on health care* (2000 $ millions)	Ontario population (thousands)	Real per-capita health care expenditures (2000 $)	Per capita health care spending deficit (94-95 minus year Y) (2000 $)	Cumulative loss in per capita health care spending, 1995-2001 (2000 $)
1994-1995	$17,683	91.2	$19,389	10,828	$1,791	0	0
1995-1996	$17,643	92.5	$19,074	10,965	$1,740	(51)	(51)
1996-1997	$17,945	93.9	$19,111	11,101	$1,722	(69)	(120)
1997-1998	$18,106	95.6	$18,939	11,260	$1,682	(109)	(229)
1998-1999	$19,427	98.9	$19,643	11,412	$1,721	(70)	(299)
1999-2000 (est.)	$20,469	100.0	$20,469	11,549	$1,772	(19)	(318)
2000-2001 (est.)	$22,288	103.0	$21,639	11,699	$1,850	59	(259)

Sources: Public Accounts of Ontario, 1995-1999, and Expenditure Estimates, 1999-2001; Statistics Canada, CANSIM Matrix P106085 (inflation projected at 3% in 2000-2001); **Canadian Institute for Health Information** (population growth projected at 1.298% 2000-2001 forward); Bill Murnighan, "Health Care Spending in Ontario," Ontario Alternative Budget Working Group, Paper No. 8, April 2000.
(*Total operating expenditures minus hospital restructuring costs.)

Spending required to make up the cumulative per capita deficit, 1994-1995 to 2000-2001: $3.0 billion percent public in 1995). In other words, by 1995 provincial public sector health expenditures in Ontario had lost all of the ground they had gained on private sector health expenditures since 1985. The balance between provincial government and private sector health expenditures has continued tipping towards the latter since then. The private sector's share of health spending in 1997 was higher in Ontario than in any other province (37.8 percent; the national average was 30.6 percent). Projections indicate that Ontario retained this distinction in 1998 and 1999.[6]

Private sector health expenditures in Ontario increased throughout the 1990s, with almost all of the increase being for drugs and the services of professionals other than physicians (i.e. mainly dental care and vision care) (see Table 3). This is consonant with the trend observed for Canada as a whole by the Canadian Institute for Health Information. After a relative decline in the private share of total health spending in the 1980s, related in part to the introduction of drug plans in a number of provinces, public spending levelled off during the 1990s as a result of government budgetary restraint. It is likely that the increased costs in Ontario are related to the introduction of user fees for prescription drugs for senior citizens and social assistance recipients, reduced public insurance coverage for vision care, as well as to the rationing of home care services. Although part of the increase in private spending is attributable to rising prices in sectors never covered by medicare, not all of it is by any means:

> Some may argue that increases in private spending happen because prices go up for things that were never covered by the pub-

Table 3
Real private health care expenditures per capita[1]
(1999 $)

Year	Hospitals	Other institutions	Physicians	Other professionals	Drugs	Other spending	Capital	Total
1994	$104	81	4	309	258	91	16	862
1995	116	80	4	324	271	94	37	926
1996	116	80	3	336	277	97	29	938
1997	115	81	3	348	316	94	19	977
1998	111	80	3	358	336	94	8	990
1999	106	80	2	366	354	92	14	1014
Change from 1994 to 1999	$2	($1)	($1)	$57	$96	$1	($2)	$152
% of private spending coming from households and private insurance[2]	40%	100%	100%	12%	81%	100%	0%	55%
New costs since 1994	$1	($1)	($1)	$7	$77	$1	$0	$84

1. Canadian Institute for Health Information, *National Health Expenditure Trends (1975-1999)*. Converted to 1999 dollars using the Health Care Price Index for Ontario, Statistics Canada.
2. Canadian Institute for Health Information, *Analytical Focus—Private Sector Spending in Canada*, 1998. The findings of this study allow the exclusion of expenditures in areas not covered by OHIP, such as dentists and certain eye care services, and the inclusion of only household and private insurance expenditures.

Source: Bill Murnighan, "Health Care Spending in Ontario," Ontario Alternative Budget Working Group, Paper No. 8, April 2000

lic system, or because of increasing charitable donations, not because of cuts to the public system. (...) 60 percent of private funding for hospitals comes from corporations and charities, while the other 40 percent comes from households and private insurance. Likewise, 81 percent of private spending on drugs (which has soared as people are sent home from hospitals quicker and sicker) comes from households and private insurance. And when you cut out the areas that were never covered by the public system (like dentists and certain eye care procedures), 12 percent of the new spending on "other professionals" can be attributed to cutbacks.[7]

The average Ontario citizen paid $84 per year more in 1999 than in 1994 in out-of-pocket health care costs. With an Ontario population of over eleven million people, this means that nearly $1 billion more is flowing every year into the private health care market from individuals' wallets and private insurance plans.[8]

Of course, such figures only show us the shift in cost that occurs when individuals are willing and able to pay more out of their own pockets, or consent to higher private insurance premiums. *What remains unquantified is the cost to those who are deterred by higher private prices and simply forego seeking treatments, services and products they previously enjoyed.* There may be many people who simply cannot afford to pay privately for their care and do without. These people do not show up in the statistics, nor do the extra costs they incur—in effort, in time, and in suffering.

It is worth noting as well that overall (public and private) health expenditures as a percentage of GDP declined in Ontario over the 1990s: 9.7 per cent in 1992 and 1993, 9.5 per cent in 1994, 9.3 per cent in 1995, 9.2 per cent in 1996, and 8.9 per cent in 1997.[9]

Re-engineering health care

Between 1995 and 1999, the Conservative government implemented many sweeping changes to health care services in Ontario, downloading some to other levels of government and reorganizing others. The two major pieces of restructuring legislation affecting health care were Bill 26, *An Act to Achieve Fiscal Savings and to Promote Economic Prosperity through Public Sector Restructuring, Streamlining and Efficiency and to Implement Other Aspects of the Government's Economic Agenda, 1996* (the provisions of which for public hospital restructuring were extended and modified by Bill 23 in December 1999), and Bill 152, the *Services Improve-*

ment Act, 1997, which implemented many of the political decisions flowing from the work of the "Who Does What" task force, notably the transfer of responsibility for financing and delivering public health programs and ambulance services to upper-tier municipalities or other agents chosen by the provincial government. Bill 67 further added to the government's ability to move swiftly, expeditiously and with fewer checks and balances, by giving the Minister of Health the power to do many things that previously required an Order in Council or a Regulation. In addition, Bill 118, the *Red Tape Reduction Act, 1997*, restructured health appeal boards and amended the health professions regulations. Bill 7, the *Labour Relations and Employment Statute Law Amendment Act, 1995* and Bill 136, which consisted of the *Public Sector Transition Stability Act, 1997*, and the *Public Sector Dispute Resolution Act, 1997*, laid the groundwork for public sector restructuring by defining the rules governing union representation and successor rights in the case of restructuring, amalgamation, contracting out, and privatization. Bill 71, the *Crown Foundations Act, 1996*, extended the status of crown foundation to many additional institutions, such as public hospitals, enhancing their ability to raise money privately through charitable giving. Bill 99, which established the *Workplace Safety and Insurance Act, 1997*, reformed workers' compensation in Ontario; Bill 127, the *Expanded Nursing Services for Patients Act, 1997*, authorized nurse-practitioners to offer a range of services previously restricted to physicians.

If there was a common theme running through most of this legislation, it was the rolling back of democracy. The provincial government did not have an electoral mandate to redistribute powers between levels of government, forcibly amalgamate municipalities and school boards, or close hospitals. Yet it passed these laws to give itself the powers to do these things swiftly and over the objections of anyone who disagreed. The constantly recurring pattern was the forcible imposition of its will on municipalities, school boards, district health councils, hospital boards, unions, and individuals. Local authorities, such as municipalities, school boards or district health councils, saw their powers and budgets slashed in the process.

The Ontario government's November 1995 *Fiscal and Economic Statement* announced a series of legislative and financial measures affecting health care. These included:
1. the formation of a Health Services Restructuring Commission "to manage and accelerate the implementation of hospital restructuring regionally and locally";
2. granting hospitals "more flexibility to generate revenues":

3. de-funding physicians' malpractice insurance;
4. introducing user fees for people receiving benefits under the Ontario Drug Benefit Plan (ODB) (see the section on user charges, below).[10]

The government immediately followed the *Fiscal Statement* with a major legislative initiative, Bill 26, the "Cost Savings and Restructuring Act," also known as the "Omnibus Bill," in November 1995. It was intended to create the legislative framework for the previously announced policy changes and restructuring measures. Bill 26 enacted or modified a large number of laws, including the Health Insurance Act, the Health Care Accessibility Act, the Ministry of Health Act, the Ontario Drug Benefit Act, the Prescription Drug Cost Regulation Act, the Public Hospitals Act, the Independent Health Facilities Act, the Regulated Health Professions Act, and the Physician Services Delivery Management Act, the Pay Equity Act, the Freedom of Information and Protection of Privacy Act, and many other laws besides. Its many provisions included the following:

1. it granted the Minister of Health sweeping powers to change the financing and operation of public hospitals, as well as the power to close or amalgamate them;
2. it made possible the establishment of private medical facilities, such as laboratories, without tendering, and removed the requirement that preference be given to Canadian non-profit organizations, thus opening the door to American for-profit businesses.
3. it granted the Minister of Health the power to dictate where in the province physicians may practice;
4. it cut pay equity payments for women and gave hospitals new powers to roll back wages;
5. it implemented drug user fees under the Ontario Drug Benefit Plan (see below);
6. it forced thousands of acute-care hospital patients waiting for a bed in a nursing home to pay a daily charge for room and board.

Slashing budgets and closing hospitals

Under Bill 26, the Harris government gave the Health Services Restructuring Commission (HSRC) a four-year mandate to restructure hospitals in Ontario and to recommend measures to restructure other parts of the health services system. The government concentrated enormous power in a few hands in order to effect huge changes.

Expenditure on hospitals has historically been by far the largest item in provincial government health expenditures—44.6 per cent in 1995. However, hospitals' share of provincial health care funding has in fact been declining steadily since the 1970s (55.5 percent in 1975, 52.0 percent in 1980, 49.9 percent in 1985, 46.5 percent in 1990, 44.6 percent in 1995, and 43.9 percent in 1998). Between 1989 and 1998, sixty-four of Ontario's hospitals were merged or closed outright. The total number of hospitals dropped from 262 to 198, a 24.4 per cent decrease.[11] Table 4 documents the decline in the number of hospital beds in Ontario between 1989 and 1998. The number of acute-care beds fell by 33.0 percent, of chronic care beds by 28.2 percent, of psychiatric beds by 16.0 percent, and of rehabilitation beds by 11.4 percent. Overall, the number of beds dropped by 30.2 percent in ten years.

In February 1999, Statistics Canada and the Canadian Institute for Health Information reported that the "rate at which Canadians stayed overnight in hospitals in the fiscal year 1996-1997 fell for the 10th straight year to a record low."[12] To a considerable extent, the decline in the number of hospitals and beds "can be traced to a sharp reduction in the hospital extended care sector and a rise in outpatient visits" driven by the imperative of containing expenditures.[13]

In Canada as a whole in 1999, the hospital discharge rate—a proxy for the number of people who receive treatment in hospital—also dropped "to its lowest level since 1961 when such data were first collected." In Ontario, the number of people discharged from hospitals decreased by 5.9 per cent between 1995-1996 and 1996-1997, while the discharge rate (the number of people discharged per 100,000 population) diminished by 7.1 per cent during the same period.[14] Table 5 shows

Table 4
Hospital beds in Ontario, 1989-1998, by year and category

Year	Acute beds	Chronic beds	Rehab beds	Psych beds	Total beds
1989-1990	33,387	11,353	2,048	2,442	49,230
1990-1991	31,891	11,451	1,975	2,365	47,682
1991-1992	29,813	11,405	1,902	2,279	45,399
1992-1993	27,929	10,913	1,926	2,228	42,996
1993-1994	26,097	10,592	1,905	2,132	40,726
1994-1995	25,386	10,325	1,853	2,138	39,702
1995-1996	24,014	9,639	1,890	2,102	37,645
1996-1997	22,084	8,678	1,875	2,098	34,735
1997-1998	22,367	8,149	1,815	2,050	34,381
% change, 1989-1998	- 33.0%	- 28.2%	- 11.4%	- 16.0%	- 30.2 %

Source: Based on data provided by the Ontario Hospital Association

Table 5
Number of cases discharged from Ontario hospitals, by year and type of hospital, 1989-1998 (hospital separations)

Year	Acute separations & psych	Chronic separations	Rehab separations (general & special)	Total separations
1989-1990	1,286,738	14,204	14,906	1,315,848
1990-1991	1,278,371	14,165	15,442	1,315,074
1991-1992	1,279,005	15,439	15,364	1,309,808
1992-1993	1,221,301	15,967	15,713	1,244,939
1993-1994	1,190,916	17,316	16,085	1,224,317
1994-1995	1,171,665	18,090	16,013	1,205,768
1995-1996	1,145,306	18,875	16850	1,181,031
1996-1997	1,074,175	18,231	17,387	1,109,793
1997-1998	1,022,477	18,653	17,862	1,058,992

Source: Based on data provided by the Ontario Hospital Association

the decline in the number of hospital separations in Ontario over the last decade.

Statistics Canada has suggested the decline in hospital discharge rates may be due to "multiple factors":

> The trend toward more frequent use of ambulatory care and day surgery, the shift from hospital to community-based services, increased emphasis on health promotion and disease prevention, improved medical technologies and treatments as well as new pharmaceuticals may have reduced the need for hospitalization or surgical intervention. In addition, all jurisdictions throughout Canada are in a process of change and transition associated with health care reform, ranging from hospital closures and administrative restructuring to the consolidation of services.[15]

There are therefore long-term trends in the form and structure of care driven by factors intrinsic to the practice of medicine. However, these do not exist in a vacuum. They are constrained and influenced by the broader fiscal and policy environment. Pressure to reduce costs is a powerful incentive for hospitals to reduce the number of in-patient admissions and to discharge patients more quickly. New technology and medical practices may make this possible; but these pressures no doubt encourage the very development of new technologies and practices. Surgical innovations have made it possible to treat people on an out-patient basis—however, the systematic development of this approach has clearly been driven by economic concerns. The biggest single cost for hospitals is wages and benefits (roughly three-quarters of hospitals' total expenses in 1998).[16] There is no doubt that hospital restructuring shifts patients from the higher- wage hospital sector to the lower-wage long-term community care sector.

Table 6
Provincial transfer payments for the operation of hospitals, 1994-2001, Ontario

Year	1994-1995	1995-1996	1996-1997	1997-1998	1998-1999	1999-2000 (est)	2000-2001 (est)
Payments (current $)	$7,316,135,963	$7,248,400,712	$7,391,337,581	$6,703,552,621	$7,077,078,570	$7,186,830,800	$7,973,721,900
Health care price index, Ontario* (2000=100)	91.2	92.5	93.9	95.6	98.9	100.0	103.0
Payments (2000 $)	$8,022,078,907	$7,836,108,878	$7,871,499,021	$7,012,084,332	$7,155,792,285	$7,186,830,800	$7,741,477,573
Hospitals' loss (1994-1995 minus year Y) (2000 $)	0	($185,970,029)	($150,579,886)	($1,009,994,575)	($866,286,622)	($835,248,107)	($280,601,334)
Hospitals' cumulative loss (2000 $)	0	($185,970,029)	($336,549,915)	($1,346,544,490)	($2,212,831,112)	($3,048,079,219)	($3,328,680,553)
Population of Ontario	10828000	10965000	11101000	11260000	11412000	11549000	11699000
Per capita provincial transfer payments to hospitals (2000 $)	$740.86	$714.65	$709.08	$622.74	$627.04	$622.29	$661.72
Loss in per capita provincial payments to hospitals (1994-1995 minus year Y)	0	($26.21)	($31.78)	($118.12)	($113.82)	($118.57)	($79.14)
Cumulative loss in per capita provincial payments to hospitals	0	($26.21)	($57.99)	($176.11)	($289.93)	($408.50)	($487.64)

*Health care price index, Statistics Canada, CANSIM Matrix P106085 (inflation projected at 3% in 2000-2001).

Source: Public Accounts of Ontario, 1994-1999, and Expenditure Estimates, 1999-2001; Canadian Institute for Health Information (population growth projected at 1.298% 2000-200 forward); Bill Murnighan, "Health Care Spending in Ontario," Ontario Alternative Budget Working Group, Paper No. 8, April 2000

The amount necessary to make up the cumulative per capita loss in hospital operating expenditures, 1994-1995 to 2000-2001: $5.7billion

The November 1995 *Fiscal and Economic Statement* announced reductions of $365 million from the hospital envelope in 1996-1997 and $435 million in 1997-1998.[17] While there were a number of spending announcements in subsequent years, notably an April 1998 government promise to spend $225 million to alleviate overcrowding in emergency wards, transfer payments from the Ministry of Health to Ontario's hospitals for operating expenditures fell dramatically between 1994 and 1999 as hospitals closed, merged and cut back (see Table 6).

The Health Services Restructuring Commission established by Bill 26 in 1996 had the mandate of finding ways of making the hospital system more efficient and cost-effective. Coming on the heels of over one billion dollars of announced reductions to hospital budgets, this could only be interpreted as a mandate to find the ways to cut that money out of the system. The HSRC ordered the closure of 45 hospitals (33 public hospitals, 6 private ones, and 6 psychiatric hospitals). Forty-four hospitals have amalgamated in fourteen new multi-site corporations. The HSRC also proposed that one hundred individual hospitals combine in eighteen networks or clusters.[18] Its rationale for closing hospitals and forcing others to amalgamate was that they contained unused space that was being heated, lit and maintained, wasting resources that ought to have been used for much needed new care.[19] Critics however pointed out that the space was not being used because the money to keep beds open had been cut. The case for reduced funding was furthermore predicated on the superior efficiency of community care—yet the community care resources still had not been created at the time the hospital budget was slashed.

However, the Health Services Restructuring Commission also found restructuring costly. Its final report noted that restructuring would cost the government $100 million more than it would save. As money spent on actually running hospitals and treating patients fell, the government set aside increasing sums to cover the costs of restructuring: $153,758,526 in 1997-1998, $248,354,216 in 1998-1999, and $512,200,000 in 1999-2000 (current dollars). Hospitals, too, were expected to bear a portion of the costs, namely "the full cost interest expense on debt incurred to fund restructuring, 15 per cent of all operating restructuring costs (e.g., severance for laid-off staff) and 30 per cent of capital restructuring."[20] In fact, while the HSRC had originally estimated the cost of its directives to hospitals at $2.1 billion, the Provincial Auditor reported that the cost might well reach nearly $4 billion (see Table 7). The Ontario Hospital Association estimates that hospitals will have to raise about $1 billion to meet their share of the government-mandated restructuring and about

$1.6 billion more for routine capital projects.[21] The money has thus flowed out of care, so that investments could be made in bricks and mortar. This is once again a transfer of money from public health care to private industry: thousands of nursing and related jobs have vanished, but developers and management consultants have done well.

Not surprisingly, hospitals are in debt; many are unable to meet their budgets (see Table 8). With accumulated deficits of around $2.3 billion, Ontario's 164 hospital corporations are in a deep crisis. The Ontario Hospital Association has called on the federal and provincial governments to invest billions of dollars in them.

After reviewing the province's funding formula for adjusting grants to hospitals, the Provincial Auditor found: "The formula has not established a clear relationship between a hospital's relative cost efficiency and its base grant. As of September 1998, approximately 34 percent of the hospitals incurring deficits were considered efficient, while 10 percent reporting surpluses were considered inefficient." Furthermore, the formula "focuses on inpatient care activities and costs, which account for approximately 60 percent of all hospital expenditures. Activities such as outpatient clinics and emergency care are excluded due to a lack of reliable statistical data."[22] In response, the Ministry of Health and Long-Term Care has said that it intends to bring in a new methodology which will address these problems. But this begs the question: if this more efficient planning tool is not in place and the Ministry has achieved the sort of hit-and-miss results reported by the Auditor, the implication is that the funding process is somewhat blind. This calls into question the whole process of restructuring.

Table 7 Summary of hospital capital costs resulting from HSRC directions, May 1999		
	HSRC's original estimate ($ billions)	Hospitals' preliminary estimate ($ billions)
Estimated cost	2.1	3.9
Potential Ministry share	1.5	2.7
Potential hospital share	0.6	1.2

Source: Provincial Auditor of Ontario, 1999

Table 8 Projected 1998/1999 hospital deficits in Ontario		
Deficit as a percentage of budget	Number of hospitals	Total deficit ($ millions)
0% to 5%	92	79
5% to 10%	20	53
More than 10%	9	104
Total	121	236

Source: Provincial Auditor of Ontario, 1999

Finally, hospital closures raise major issues of social justice. The chances of being hospitalized are inversely proportional to one's income. Many studies have established correlations between poverty, inequality and ill health.[23] In Ontario, hospital admission rates for people in poor health "are nearly twice as high among poor people as they are among non-poor people."[24] This is not true in the United States, where universal medicare does not exist and people living in poverty are deterred from using hospitals by prohibitive out-of-pocket costs. The implications of closing hospitals are clear. In Ontario, the rich and the poor alike can receive comprehensive care fully paid for by the public purse in the hospital. Outside of hospital, however, the situation is far dicier. Home care is rationed (see next chapter)—private home care, at $14 or $15 an hour (for a homemaker, a private nurse would cost much more), is out of most people's reach. Community care may indeed often be preferable to the hospital from both a social and a medical point of view. But until it is universally available as an insured service to all Ontarians, governments should not be closing hospitals. This was in fact the position of the head of the government's own Health Services Restructuring Commission, Dr. Duncan Sinclair:

> Dr. Sinclair agreed that [community] services must be in place at the time the [hospital] cuts are implemented. In fact, the government agreed to this as a condition for the Commission's work, and the Commission has threatened resignation at government delays in putting alternatives in place. Dr. Sinclair is convinced the government will hold to their bargain and implement "reinvestments" before closing hospitals and hospital beds.[25]

Unfortunately, Dr. Sinclair appears to have been mistaken.

Restructuring hospitals

Hospitals have responded to cutbacks throughout the 1990s by implementing their own internal restructuring and re-engineering plans. As a recent study puts it:

> These financial challenges led to the acceleration of the changes in acute care hospitals, including efforts to downsize, re-engineer, and restructure service delivery. Administrative cost-containment strategies used included early retirement, outsourcing of work, increased use of temporary and part-time workers and of volunteers, decentralizing units and services, pay cuts, etc. Work re-design or re-engineering to reduce costs was embraced as a cost-saving measure that could maintain quality of care and improve job design.[26]

A central feature of hospital restructuring has been the attempt by hospitals "to adapt a business-like approach to health care," by resorting to "new management techniques such as total quality management, re-engineering, and program-management re-organization among others."[27]

A study of 15 Ontario hospitals by two professors from McMaster University's Degroot School of Business found that the hospitals' chief executive officers were enthusiastic about this new direction. Interestingly, though, the change has not come without resistance at various levels: "in the two hospitals where formal quality programs were not in use, the reason given was that hospital staff, particularly physicians, found such programs to be too 'businesslike' and inappropriate for the hospital because they believed quality to be an inherent requirement of health care and felt such a program called their practice into question."[28] Similarly, the Provincial Auditor reports:

> In 1998, the Ministry retained consultants to assess the effectiveness of the existing hospital operating plan process in addressing accountability. In their report, the consultants noted a lack of mutual understanding about accountability relationships. For example, the consultants noted that while the Ministry believes that hospitals are accountable to it for the expenditure of public funds, hospitals feel that they are accountable to their communities and patients and that the Ministry is primarily a payment agency.[29]

Clearly, an intolerable situation! The consultants consequently recommended that the Ministry develop an accountability framework to govern its relations with hospitals and "redesign hospital operating plans to reflect and support the new framework." In response, the Ministry set up a task force made up of "representatives from the Ministry, the Ontario Hospital Association, hospital management and other stakeholder groups."[30] As a recent report has drily observed: "Financial goals are often more central to decision-making than quality of care."[31]

Hospital re-engineering has taken a number of forms. Like factories operating in a regime of post-fordist "lean production," most of the hospitals in Chan and Lynn's study "had adopted just-in-time (JIT) inventory systems and paperless material management," and joined with other hospitals in "consortium purchasing agreements to reduce materials purchasing and administration costs." Some had hired management consulting firms specialized in restructuring and merging hospitals, such as APM Inc., to advise them on how to reduce costs and re-organize their operations. Many had decided to reduce their administrative expenses by contracting out their "hospitality and housekeeping services," i.e. cleaning and food preparation, or "by sharing such services with other hospitals."[32] The London Health Sciences Centre, for example, has outsourced a whole range of functions: "ServiceMaster Healthcare Management Services was contracted to provide integrated support services, Clintar to manage grounds maintenance, Data Business Forms to install and run the printing department with digital technology, U.S. Turbine and Laidlaw to run the energy and waste management systems, and SERCA and Summit to jointly operate the food services department."[33] The "outsourcing" of these services provides significant opportunities for commercial enterprises. A number of large corporations heve been active in this field, such as Marriott International, Sodexho (which has recently merged with Marriott), ServiceMaster, Aramark, and Cara. Outsourcing has become increasingly attractive to corporations as hospitals amalgamate or form networks, and integrate their operations.

Entering into "public-private partnerships" for laboratory services has also been a popular strategy among hospital administrations.[34] In fact, the integration of laboratory services in Ontario began a decade ago. A 1992 review of the laboratory sector by the Ministry of Health criticized the lack of co-ordination between private, public and hospital laboratories, blaming it for inefficient use of health care resources. It called for the technological, legislative, management and planning conditions of laboratory integration to be put in place. The Ministry of Health has been driving laboratory reform through its Laboratory Secretariat and through the Health Services Restructuring Commission.

The big story behind integration is the squeeze on hospitals and their laboratories on the one hand, and the consolidation of a private-sector oligopoly on the other. Although private laboratories started many years ago as small operations funded by the private insurance industry and serving physicians' offices, the situation has evolved to the point where "[t]hree major private laboratory companies have close to 90 percent of the market."[35] These are MDS Inc., Dynacare, and Canadian Medical Laboratories.[36] They have pursued an expansionary strategy familiar in other industries as well, creating large automated facilities that can process huge volumes of specimens, thus lowering unit prices. However, "[s]ince a key factor to individual laboratory viability is the ratio of volume of testing to the number of testing laboratories, competition has extended beyond the private sector into the hospital sector."[37]

Hospital laboratories, meanwhile have been squeezed by falling hospital budgets. The attractiveness of the public sector to private firms as a source of greater service volume and the desperate financial situation of public hospitals have pushed both sides towards "public/private partnerships." Sunnybrook Hospital in Toronto joined with Dynacare Laboratories to form SDL Laboratories. Sunnybrook's Chief Executive Officer was quoted as saying: "It'll be a whole new revenue system for us. We have zero percent increase from the government and we're looking for new revenues."[38] The hospital hoped that its partnership with Dynacare would bring in revenue from new business with other Ontario hospitals and the United States. Similarly, the Toronto Hospital formed a partnership with MDS Inc. in 1995 to use the Autolab technology MDS had developed. This technology has been described as a "fully automated computerized process management system [using] robotics for handling specimens and carrying out testing."[39]

Public laboratories operate at a disadvantage. Where private laboratories bill OHIP on a fee-for-service basis, public laboratories must make do with whatever they get under the province's block funding to the hospitals. This means that they do not have the means or the incentive to deal with higher volumes of service, especially out-patient work, and that they have not always the means to invest in new technology or facilities.[40] Furthermore, public laboratories must deal with more complicated and less profitable tasks:

> In addition to the routine work they carry out, [public laboratories] are also responsible for carrying out extremely specialized, complicated, non-routine work. This requires a lot of effort, skilled technologists, and often involves high-cost equipment. The demand on an hour-by-hour basis for this equipment is not necessarily that great—it often stands idle for much of the day and operates in expensive short runs. Nevertheless, in many instances, it is only this high-cost technologically advanced equipment that can provide the proper detection and diagnosis of life-threatening illnesses.

Private laboratories tend to avoid this extremely specialized, complicated, non-routine work in favour of the high-volume, less-expensive routine laboratory work.[41] Private laboratories have been able to skim the cream of the business, leaving the less lucrative work to the public sector.

With dwindling government funding for hospitals, business has flowed to private laboratories. The fee-for-service model has in fact led to escalating costs in the private sector, inciting the provincial government to cap private laboratory billing:

> In December 1993, the Ministry of Health signed a three-year agreement with the Ontario Association of Medical Laboratories

in order to reduce payments to private laboratories by 8.9 percent over a three-year period. Expenditures to private laboratories had been increasing by about 15 percent a year throughout the 1980s. These reductions were to bring expenditures from the 1992-1993 high of $456 million to a maximum of $415 million by 1995-1996. The ceiling for 1993-1994 was set at $433 million but payments soared to $480 million.[42]

In 1998, the government negotiated a new cap on the business of $425 million, with scheduled increases of 1.5 percent in each of 1998-1999 and 1999-2000. However, this was superseded by a further agreement between the Ministry of Health and Long-Term Care and the industry's representative, the Ontario Association of Medical Laboratories. Under this agreement, private laboratories received a one-time retroactive payment of $26.6 million for 1998-1999, and a 1999-2000 global envelope of $458 million.[43]

The 1998 plan to cap rising prices led to severe criticism and a court challenge. Essentially, the $425 million envelope was to be divided among firms on the basis of their respective 1996 market shares. *Globe and Mail* columnist Terence Corcoran described the plan as "bizarre":

> First, the regulation forces all firms in the industry to retreat to the individual market share positions each held more than two years ago—effectively taking away business from the successful and awarding it to firms that failed to grow. Then, the government intends to pay the labs for their 1998 work only on the basis of the 1996 market share. The effect here would be to force the winning firms to send money back to the government.[44]

The federal Competition Bureau was highly critical of the plan. It indicated that Ontario was suffering from "an oversupply of medical lab services, or at least an oversupply relative to what the province currently believes it needs or wants to pay for."[45] But this excess capacity is the result of government policies which have encouraged the private sector labs at the expense of their more efficient public sector counterparts.

The driving force behind laboratory privatization is supposedly the private sector's superior efficiency. Yet, a number of studies conducted over the last two decades indicate that private laboratory services in fact cost more.[46] It has been inferred from these studies that OHIP's laboratory costs could be reduced by $200-250 million a year, if the public sector were to take over the business.[47] This is roughly the same amount that senior citizens and social assistance recipients are obliged to pay in user fees for prescription drugs (see below).

"Rationalizing" the workforce

Between 1995 and 1998, the number of hospital workers in Ontario dropped from 154,000 to 127,000. Most of the roughly 27,000 workers who left the workplace did so as a result of lay-offs and early retirement.[48] The number of nurses working in Ontario dropped by 3.8 percent between 1994 and 1999, according to a conservative estimate (from 107,313 to 103,363). Most of this decline was among registered nurses (from 82,069 to 78,174), although the number of registered practical nurses also dropped. The decrease has been sharpest among nurses holding full-time positions—7.5 per cent for registered nurses (42,328 in 1994 to 39,134 in 1999) and 4 percent for registered practical nurses (12,365 in 1994 to 11,869 in 1999). Fully 36 percent of Ontario nurses worked part-time in 1999, while 14 percent held casual positions.[49]

There was also a significant shift in nursing employment from hospitals and public homes for the aged—5,590 registered nurses and 1,430 registered practical nurses—to private nursing homes, retirement homes and home care between 1994 and 1999—1,591 registered nurses and 1,875 registered practical nurses (see Table 9). There are reports that patients are having to resort to hiring private nurses to look after their needs whil in hospital, or to rely on family and friends to do so.[50]

Studies have linked downsizing to higher work loads and stress, worsening morale, lower job security, and increasing sick leave and absenteeism. There are indications that the changes involving nurses have had a detrimental impact on patient care: "Hospitals with a higher percentage of RNs and higher staffing ratios of nurse to patient had lower mortality rates."[51] A 1997 study conducted by the Ivey School of Business for the Ontario Hospital Association found "lower levels of cleanliness, reduced patient supervision, increased employee stress, and less nursing time per patient" in Ontario hospitals.[52] Indeed, after a year of restructuring at one hospital:

Table 9 Nursing jobs gained or lost between 1994 and 1999		
Sector	Registered nurses	Registered practical nurses
Hospitals	-4,997	-1,328
Public homes for the aged	-593	-102
Private nursing homes	727	890
Retirement homes	212	349
Home care	652	636

Source: RNAO/RPNAO—*Report on Nursing Recruitment and Retention in Ontario*

> The morale of staff and their trust in the organization decreased markedly. The changes introduced produced more negative feelings about the hospital as a place to work and led to a deterioration of the relationship between the organization and its employees. A recent study of nurses showed that organizational and professional job satisfaction were strong predictors of process measures of quality of care. (...) The concerns raised by staff in this longitudinal study are congruent with qualitative research regarding the effects of changes in Ontario hospitals. Nicholson suggests that downsizing shatters security and trust, which are not readily rebuilt. Our data suggest that large-scale re-engineering in a brief period of time may have similar effects.[53]

A major study published in the Canadian Medical Association Journal indicated that "reported errors" had increased substantially between 1992 and 1997:

> Misadventures rose from 18 to 30 per 10,000 for in-patients and 5.2 to 11.6 for day surgeries. Complications rose from 330 to 500 per 10,000 for in-patients and 65.2 to 95.1 per 10,000 for day surgeries. Adverse drug reactions rose from 104 to 162 per 10,000 for in-patients and 8.1 to 10.8 per 10,000 for day surgeries. The authors conclude that the only plausible sources of the change are either a change in rates and methods of reporting, or deterioration in the quality of care delivered.[54]

Nursing staff shortages in hospitals and the shift from full-time to part-time employment for nurses can reduce the continuity of care and diffuse accountability for patient care. Such reduction and diffusion has been shown to be linked to increased infection rates among hospital patients. Coroners' juries have recently "pinpointed the need for an appropriate number or 'safe ratio' of nurses in emergency wards and other hospital units, as well as the need for trained professionals (such as nurses) to assess and triage patients, and for nurses to receive ongoing education and training."[55]

Faced with concern voiced by the nurses, the Minister of Health established the Nursing Task Force in September 1998 "to examine nursing services in Ontario, to identify how changes in the profession have affected the delivery of health care services, and to recommend how the province's health system can be improved through nursing services." In February 1999, the Task Force presented a report calling on the provincial government to:

- invest $375 million annually "to create additional permanent front line nursing positions before the Year 2000," with $125 million of that money to be spent "no later than March 31, 1999."
- amend relevant legislation to ensure a "meaningful" part for nurses in "decisions that affect patient care on both a corporate and an operational level."
- "invest an additional $1 million annually for research to support a comprehensive nursing resource database."
- work with nurses and employers to redress inequities in the remuneration of nurses in the home care sector.[56]

The provincial government made a public commitment to address the report's recommendations. In March 1999, Minister Witmer annnounced that $130 million would be invested to "enable hospitals to employ over 3,300 new permanent nurses (full and part-time) over the next year."[57] The Ministry of Health further stated that it would, by 1999/2000, "have invested a total of $375 million in nursing, with annual increases, e.g., $109 million in 2000/2001, making a total of $484 million for that year." It claimed that these investments would "create over 12,100 full and part-time permanent positions over the 1998/99 to 2000/01 period."[58]

The government's announcements were the object of criticism from several quarters. The *Toronto Star* questioned Minister Witmer's promise to spend $375 million to (re)hire 10,000 nurses, asking whether these 10,000 included the 7,900 hirings already promised.[59] The *Star* pointed out that the "government uses five different sets of numbers to describe last April's $1.2 billion announcement on community and long-term care—7,900 jobs over eight years, 7,900 over six years, 7,400, 5,100, and 11,850," while the March 1999 response to the Nursing Task Force spoke of 12,100 "new nursing jobs." From this, the *Star* suggested, should be deducted 1,900 jobs already created, 5,250 community care and long-term-care nurses included in the previously announced 7,900, 200 hired in 1998 by the Workplace Safety and Insurance Board, and 3,700 nursing jobs lost as a result of hospital closings. This would leave 1,050 new jobs. However, the *Star* pointed out, Premier Harris had announced the expenditure of $39,000 per nurse to cover salary, benefits and payroll costs—the jobs could therefore only be part-time. The *Star*'s conclusion:

> So, we are not watching new health care being created. We're watching Harris laundering his old promises so that—through this "special account"—Ottawa ends up paying for them. This isn't about health care, in other words. It's a refinancing—to free

up $1.5 billion so Harris can cut taxes at federal expense—at nurses' and patients' expense, too.[60]

Barb Wahl, the head of the Ontario Nurses Association, also criticized the government's promise, claiming that the money granted to hospitals to hire nurses might well end up being used to cover a part of the hospitals' massive debt. Hilary Short, vice-president of the Ontario Hospital Association, reportedly confirmed that, because of their ongoing operating deficits, hospitals had no fund with which to meet the promise of hiring new nurses.[61] An April 2000 joint report by the Registered Nurses Association and the Registered Practical Nurses Association warned that Ontario would be needing between 60,000 and 90,000 new nurses by the year 2011.[62]

Private fund-raising

In addition to outright closures, outsourcing and layoffs, cuts affected hospitals in other ways as well. For example, the government provided Toronto hospitals with $600,000 in late 1998 to run MRI machines. However, the hospitals had to buy the machines themselves, at a cost of $2.5 million per unit. Furthermore, each one costs $1 million a year to run. The hospitals were faced with $3.4 million in additional operational costs. To top it all off, the government removed the "extra-hours funding" it had previously provided to enable the hospitals to run existing MRI machines twenty-four hours a day. This placed hospitals in the position of having to rent out the machines to private customers—insurance companies, the Workplace Safety and Insurance Board, veterinarians, professional athletes—in order to be able to pay for their operation.[63] Private payers thus get to head the queue, leaving everyone else to await their turn—two-tier medicine driven by government under-funding.

Hospitals increasingly rely on private sector funding, although the lion's share of their budgets still comes out of provincial government coffers. Hospitals have also gone in for franchising, making deals with companies such as Tim Horton's or Second Cup. Other hospitals agreed to test new information technology or management systems, on the understanding that the companies developing them would pay a share of the royalties and offer cheaper rates for them if those products went to market and were successful. Hospitals are also selling advertising space on their walls, renting out their equipment, and raising money through charitable fund-raising. The Toronto Hospital even issued $281 million worth of bonds to pay for new capital spending.

As they slashed social and cultural spending in the 1990s, federal and provincial governments proclaimed the necessity of making it easier for worthy causes to raise money for themselves privately, by way of charitable giving. In the 1994, 1996 and 1997 federal budgets, Canada's Finance Minister Paul Martin altered the conditions governing charitable tax credits to encourage giving, especially among very wealthy potential donors. Revenue Canada had previously granted individuals charitable tax credits for gifts equivalent to a maximum of 20 percent of their net income. The 1996 budget had raised this to 50 percent. Donors could receive charitable tax credits for gifts worth up to 100 percent of their net income if they were donating money to the crown (this was lowered to 75 percent in the 1997 federal budget).

Ontario's *Crown Foundation Act, 1996* had the same purpose. With Bill 71, Ontario Finance Minister Ernie Eves extended the status of crown foundation to a number of institutions[64] which had already enjoyed charitable status, but could now hope to attract much larger gifts than before.[65]

> The policy appears to be the harbinger of a new approach to the funding of public institutions. The establishment of Crown foundations by governments of different political persuasions facilitates the acquisition of major gifts and signifies a recognition that novel ways have to be found for the funding of public and semi-public institutions. Matching or Challenge Funds reinforce the advantages provided by the Crown foundations by encouraging the various stakeholders in society, particularly the corporate community and research councils, to invest in the development of public institutions. Donors, individuals as well as corporate, will be expected to play a greater role in supporting universities, hospitals, museums, libraries.[66]

The government said that it could no longer afford to increase funding for such institutions, but could "give them the legislative tools to raise additional funds by encouraging public donations."[67] However, the mere fact that such donations are expected indicates a belief by the government that the money *is* available in the community.[68] The government could raise that money in taxes and spend it on hospitals and cultural institutions. Instead, it foregoes that potential tax revenue and encourages individuals to spend the money philanthropically by offering to reduce their actual taxes if they do so. In effect, it spends money, but in a different way—this is known as a "tax expenditure."[69] *In effect, by leaving the choice of how the money should be spent to individual taxpayers, the government privatizes crucial decisions on public expenditures.* It may seem democratic to leave it up to individual citizens to make such decisions—but it is not, when done in this form. Decisions are made by millions of individuals acting alone, like in the marketplace, rather than on the basis of a collective decision-making process based on a thorough, open, and rational discussion involving all citizens.[70]

Long-term care

In addition to home care, long-term-care facilities have become attractive to governments as alternatives to chronic-care hospitals: care in the latter is funded at $200 per day, while in the former it is funded at $90 per day.[71] According to 1998 Ontario government figures, there were 498 nursing homes and homes for the aged in the province, serving 57,000 people. They included 326 nursing homes serving 31,261 people, 102 municipal homes for the aged serving 16,689 people, and 70 charitable homes for the aged serving 8,976 people. Some of these institutions were run by the public sector, some by the private for-profit sector, and some by the non-profit sector.[72]

Although all long-term facilities serve similar populations, must conform to the same standards, and are all funded the same way by the provincial government, they are divided into different categories and are governed by separate legislation for historical reasons. Nursing homes are licensed by the Ministry of Health under the *Nursing Homes Act*. About 90 percent of them are run by for-profit firms, while the rest are non-profit corporations. Municipal homes for the aged are operated by municipalities under the *Homes for the Aged and Rest Homes Act*, by virtue of which every municipality not in a territorial district must establish and run such a facility either alone or in common with other municipalities. Charitable Homes for the Aged are operated by charitable organizations under the *Charitable Institutions Act*.

Wages and benefits represent the largest single expenditure item for long-term care facilities. There are significant differences among them in this respect. Homes for the aged tend to employ more nurses than nursing homes, while the latter are more likely to employ more health care aides. Salary levels are also very different. In municipal homes for the aged, nurses earned an average of $64,000 per year in 1995, while charitable and nursing homes paid an average of $56,000. For health care aides, the figures were $46,000 and $33,000 respectively.[73] This is true of other sectors that provide care. For example, municipal child care facilities pay significantly higher wages than non-profit or for-profit facilities. It is significant in this regard that the public homes for the aged have lost hundreds of nursing positions, while private nursing homes have gained hundreds more. Between 1994 and 1999, public homes for the aged lost 593 RNs and 102 RPNs, while private nursing homes gained 727 RNs and 890 RPNs (see Table 9).Unfortunately, this increase in nursing numbers does not in itself tell us anything about whether care is improving at all in those institutions. What it does tell us is that money is flowing from the higher-wage to the lower-wage sectors.

In March 1996, Health Minister Jim Wilson announced a $170 million increase in home care expenditures for 1997. Significantly, this was accompanied by a cut of up to 30 per cent in funding for nursing homes and homes for the aged, mainly among charitable and municipal homes for the aged, and a funding increase of up to 15 per cent for other institutions, mainly in the private for-profit sector. It was also expected that funding would shift from institutional to community care.[74] The new funding formula was to be based on an assessment of the individual needs of the patients in each institution. However, those needs have grown considerably:

> Long-term care facilities serve residents who have much more complex needs than ever before. The resident classification data reveal this trend. Between 1993 and 1996, there was an increase of almost 4,000 residents classified in the top three levels of care acuity, and a drop of almost 2,500 in the two least acute categories. The sudden change in resident acuity has placed significant stress on residents and on care providers, and has strained the resources within the sector. Other indicators of need, such as the Case Mix Measure, have increased sharply in the long-term care sector—9 percent between 1993 and 1999 alone. This problem can be expected to increase as more chronic care hospitals close under the directions of the Health Services Restructuring Commission.[75]

Acceptance criteria for chronic-care patients have also become more rigid. Many patients in institutions such as Ottawa's St.Vincent's Hospital, a chronic care institution, would no longer be accepted today. They would instead be sent to long-term-care facilities, where they would receive a lower standard of care, with only a small part of the medical services available in chronic care. The medical chief of chronic care at St. Vincent's said:

> [In the past] we could take a little bit [of the financial resources] away from the lighter patients to give it to the heavier patients. And now, the more heavy patients we get, we're absolutely running out. [The newer patients have much greater needs than their

predecessors.] Now you admit someone who has a feeding tube, wounds that need to be dressed and changed so many times a day, and all sorts of therapy needs. So you're replacing a patient who was light care, and we're not getting more money, we're getting less money, but every day we bring in someone with heavier needs than the one that left. That is our fundamental problem.[76]

In spite of the growing acuity of the case mix, the government abandoned a guarantee that each patient in a nursing home would receive a minimum of 2.25 hours of personal care a day, as well as the requirement that nursing homes have at least one registered nurse on the premises around the clock.[77] The Provincial Auditor had recommended that the government eliminate the 2.25 hour floor, saying that the number was not based on any research evidence.[78] Yet, as Pat Armstrong and Hugh Armstrong point out:

"Long-term care facilities now have to deal with a patient population of whom 60 percent require heavy care, estimated to be 3.5 hours per day or more," and this is before the transfer of all those patients forced out of chronic care and acute-care hospitals. Most of this population is female. Indeed, it could be said that long-term care is care for women by women. In 1997, almost three quarters of the residents in long-term care facilities were widowed women between the ages of 80 and 89. Most had multiple health problems, with 60 percent suffering from mental disorders and the same proportion from incontinence. Close to half had circulatory diseases and 46 percent had musculoskeletal disabilities. The majority required "considerable supervision and assistance with activities of daily living." They took on average four or more medications each day and nearly a third required special treatments ordered by their physicians and provided by nursing staff, ranging from catheters to ostomies to oxygen.[79]

Not surprisingly, then, there were reports by staff and patients that staffing levels and service standards had fallen to unacceptable levels in some institutions: "A study of the long-term-care sector carried out by the Ministry of Health found that 75 per cent of staff reported having inadequate time to meet residents' care requirements, with the majority of staff requiring more time to complete required care."[80] The drop in standards of care led to protests and demonstrations at some nursing homes.[81]

In March 1997, none of the $170 million had yet been spent. Minister Wilson re-announced the expenditure of some of it, which may in fact already have been money already promised by the Rae government. The Metropolitan Toronto Homecare Program pointed out that a study done for the latter in 1993 had projected that Toronto would need $70 million a year at least to reach the provincial average. In the meantime, demand had risen: between 1994 and 1997, 1,400 beds had closed in Metro hospitals and demand for home care had soared by 67 per cent.[82]

In August 1997, the Canadian Union of Public Employees and the Service Employees International Union released the results of a survey of 2,800 care providers. Ninety-four per cent of the respondents noted a "significant decline" in the quality of nursing care over the preceding year. Nearly 80 per cent reported that the units in which they worked were short-staffed, while workloads were increasing and patients' needs were becoming greater. The report blamed these problems on two main factors: the shift of sicker patients from hospitals and chronic-care facilities into nursing homes and homes for the aged; and the elimination by the government of minimum standards of care.[83]

In the face of growing public concern about the crisis of home and community care, and the government's apparent failure to reinvest the savings from hospital closures into home care, the 1998 Throne Speech promised massive investment in long-term care. In April 1998, with much fanfare, Health Minister Elizabeth Witmer announced that the government would spend $1.2 billion over eight years to enhance long-term care in Ontario, in particular by creating 20,000 new spaces in nursing homes and homes for the aged. (In March 1999, Premier Harris promised that the 20,000 spaces would be provided by 2004, rather than 2006, thanks to increased federal transfers under the Canada Health and Social Transfer.[84]) Six-hundred-and-two million dollars would be spent on operating new hursing homes and homes for the aged, as well as enhancing services in existing long-term-care facilities, $551 million would be spent on improved community care "including visiting nurses, therapists and homemakers, day programs and Meals on Wheels," and $96 million a year would be invested in the construction and renovation of nursing homes. The government predicted that the new money would generate 70,000 new jobs—27,500 "new front-line health jobs," of which 7,900 would be for registered nurses and registered practical nurses (see the section on nurses above), while 19,600 would be for homemakers, health care aides and other workers. The government also promised that its building plans would create 42,500 construction jobs.[85] As *The Globe and Mail* pointed out: "Competition to build new old-age homes is open to both private-sector and non-profit agencies, all of which will be eligible for special financing and cost-sharing programs for construction and operating funding that averages out to about $95 a day per resident, depending on the level of care needed."[86]

The government's announcement met with scepticism from the opposition, which noted that the Ministries of Health and Long-Term Care had yet to spend $170 million earmarked for long-term care in 1996:

> What is more, what you are doing is moving people from the publicly funded, publicly accountable health care service into the privatized area—privatized within the home, privatized within the community—in a way in which we know you will encourage large corporations to take on that care. We've all observed what you did with the CCACs—putting things out to tender, basing it on a market basis—which means that our public health care dollars, my tax dollars, are going to end up in the pockets of big corporate managers, big corporate companies, not put into the care of my community. I resent that and I think the people of Ontario will resent that as they watch you encouraging that privatization.[87]

But what if big companies offer better service? The evidence suggests this is not the case, as Hugh Armstrong and Pat Armstrong point out:

> The simple answer was offered to Cabinet by the Conservative Health Minister in 1969: "They are concerned about one thing only, making as much money as possible and giving as little as possible in return to the patients (...) the sooner this is gotten into on a public basis, the sooner we will be able to provide good quality health care for this segment of the population." He came to this conclusion after the government had tried setting standards, requiring reporting and developing other forms of regulation. In 1990, Vera Ingrid Tarman came to a similar conclusion after comparing the for-profit and not-for-profit homes. Although she recognized that the not-for-profits were far from perfect, she found that they "have provided care that better meets the criteria of access, accountability and quality of care." By contrast, "the ambition to provide efficient services and incorporate a profit has been at the expense of providing reasonable levels of health care."[88]

For example, an editorial in the *Ottawa Citizen* reported that provincial health officials "found 22 violations of provincial standards—everything from improper drug storage and a lack of privacy to filthy wheelchairs and unappetizing food" when they inspected a commercially operated nursing home in Ottawa in January 1999.[89] Yet, when the Ontario government pledged money in October 1998 to open 320 new long-term beds in Ottawa-Carleton, 270 of these were to be operated by private firms.

The announcement that the province would invest $1.2 billion in long-term care was also greeted with caution by the Ontario Nurses Association, which pointed out that thousands of nurses' jobs had been eliminated since 1993, that enrolment in university and college nursing programs had declined by 12 percent between 1990 and 1995, and that new nursing jobs in community care offered neither salaries, working hours and conditions, nor job security on a par with hospital employment.[90]

It rapidly became clear as well that the announced expansion of long-term care would be insufficient to meet the expected demand. Ottawa-Carleton Regional Councillor Alex Munter pointed out that the 1,313 new long-term beds promised for Ottawa-Carleton over the next eight years would not suffice, since 1,643 people were already on a waiting list for such beds.[91] Across Ontario in late 1998, there were 17,000 people on the waiting list for the 20,000 beds due only by 2006.[92]

In spite of the succession of promises, transfer payments from the province to long-term-care facilities, like health care spending in general, declined between 1994-1995 and 1997-1998, when measured in constant dollars and on a per capita basis. While 1998-1999 witnessed an increase over the two preceding years and spending was projected to rise in 1999-2000 and 2000-2001, it still lagged behind 1994-1995 and 1995-1996 (see Table 10). The cumulative per capita loss of spending on long-term care since 1994-1995 stood at $906 in 2000.

Ambulance services

Because of an absence of standards in the sector, the provincial government took over responsibility for ambulance services in the 1960s, replacing the "funeral homes, municipalities, hospitals, gas stations and a

Table 10
Provincial transfer payments for long-term-care residential services, 1994-2001

Year	Transfer payment ($ current)	Health care price index (2000=100)	Transfer payment (2000 $)	Population 75 and over	Ratio $/75+ population	Per capita spending deficit	Cumulative per capita spending deficit
1994-1995	$1,146,312,000	91.2	$1,256,921,053	530,256	$2,370	0	0
1995-1996	$1,167,745,000	92.5	$1,262,427,027	551,058	$2,291	(79)	(79)
1996-1997	$1,150,789,000	93.9	$1,225,547,391	574,154	$2,135	(235)	(314)
1997-1998	$1,212,840,000	95.6	$1,268,661,088	597,604	$2,123	(247)	(561)
1998-1999	$1,345,876,000	98.9	$1,360,845,298	621,575	$2,189	(181)	(742)
1999-2000 (est)	$1,426,053,100	100.0	$1,426,053,100	646,438	$2,206	(164)	(906)
2000-2001 (est)	$1,574,947,100	103.0	$1,529,074,854	672,295	$2,274	(96)	(1002)

Source: Public Accounts of Ontario, 1994-1999, and Expenditure Estimates, 1999-2001; Statistics Canada, CANSIM Matrix P106085 (inflation projected at 3% in 2000-2001); Statistics Canada CANSIM Matrix (growth of population 75 years and over estimated at 4% for 1999-2000 and 2000-2001)

variety of private businesses" which had previously offered the service ("Vehicles used as ambulances varied from pickup trucks to station wagons, equipment varied from provider to provider, and attendant training ranged from none at all to advanced first aid."[93]) The province passed the *Ambulance Act*, as a result of which proper standards, equipment and communications networks were put in place. Furthermore, regulations issued in 1975 "established qualifications for ambulance employees, financial and reporting requirements, and general operating procedures in order to standardize services across the province."[94] The province created a network of Central Ambulance Communications Centres (CACCs—not to be confused with CCACs, Community Care Access Centres) throughout the province; these centres "monitor the location and availability of ambulances to ensure the best possible response times and the most efficient use of vehicles."[95]

The resulting integrated, province-wide system ensured not only coordination of different services, but also adequate training of ambulance personnel. Services were delivered by the Ministry of Health, hospitals and private operators. The latter did not, however, "act as true entrepreneurs," but were considered "crown agents for the purposes of collective bargaining."[96] The ambulance system thus set up was a public, non-profit system. That having been said, ambulance services involve a co-payment of $45 per journey.[97] Furthermore, "ambulance service is not an insured service if it is not medically necessary."[98] Use of the service in such conditions entails payment of a $240 fee.[99]

Early in its first mandate, the Harris government created a commission headed by David Crombie to propose ways of "disentangling" the responsibilities and missions of the provincial and municipal governments. On May 1, 1997, the government announced a package of reforms partly based on the recommendations of this so-called "Who Does What" commission. A key part of the reform was the redistribution of financial responsibilities between the two tiers of government. The province assumed the full burden of paying for education, removing it entirely from the property tax base. In exchange, it assigned the municipalities new responsibilities. Some of this was enshrined in law by Bill 152, the *Services Improvement Act*, which among other things (e.g., child care, social housing, sewage inspections) transferred entire responsibility for funding land ambulance and public health services to municipal governments. A provincial government backgrounder announcing the change said that this would allow "the government to move ahead with changes to provide better services at lower cost to tax payers."[100]

Under Bill 152, every "upper-tier" (i.e. regional or county) municipality was to take on full responsibility for *funding* land ambulance services on January 1, 1998, and for *delivering* or *contracting for* those services on January 1, 2000. The two-year interval was meant to afford municipalities a transition period during which to plan how best to deliver the service. The province required them by September 30, 1999 to select one of three options: direct delivery of the service itself, contracting out of the service to an existing ambulance operator, or issuing a Request for Proposals (RFP) to solicit bids from potential operators. The province, meanwhile, was to remain responsible for integrating the ambulance system with the rest of the health care system; setting legislative and other standards, including best practices, guidelines and protocols; licensing services and staff. The province also indicated that it wished to continue operating the CACCs.

The province subsequently amended this plan by giving municipalities an extra year, until January 1, 2001, to take over full control of ambulance services, and by assuming 50 percent of ambulance costs as of January 1, 1999.

Critics of Bill 152 pointed out that it threatened to return Ontario to the incoherent, inefficient and inequitable situation that had existed before the *Ambulance Act*. They pointed out that David Crombie himself, the Chair of the Who Does What commission, had advised against downloading ambulance services to the municipalities, on the grounds that property taxes are not an appropriate base for social services. They worried that some municipalities would be able to afford outstanding service, while others would not. The Ontario Hospital Association questioned the wisdom of downloading, pointing out that it flew in the face of the official plan of integrating the health care system, while also further entangling the two levels of government, rather than disentangling them. The municipalities for their part opposed the plan, expressing concern that it exposed them to a new source of potentially escalating costs, without giving them the means to contain them, at a time when the province had already substantially cut its transfers to lower levels of government. The municipalities said that service standards and demand for the service would be out of their control:

> Municipalities are concerned that they are out of the loop at the present time when decisions are made about the use of ambulances. At the moment it is the attending physicians, the hospitals and dispatch that order ambulances for facility transfers. There is no cost control incentive in the system... Municipal officials were still concerned that hospitals would continue to order ambulances

for inappropriate cases because of convenience and cost-avoidance.[101]

The fear of having costs shifted to them by hospitals may or may not have been legitimate. The key point here is that such a fear would not arise in a truly integrated health care system in which a single tier of government would be responsible for all service delivery. Because of its broader and plural tax base, the provincial government ought to assume full responsibility for this system, not local government.

The Ontario Public Service Employees Union and the Canadian Union of Public Employees, for their part, voiced concern at the potential for privatization inherent in the options presented to municipalities by the province. The contracting-out and RFP options would open the door to for-profit ambulance services in Ontario. Some municipalities might choose such a path, believing in the private sector's ability to provide a more efficient service at a lower price. However, achieving such results, while still realizing a profit acceptable to the owners or shareholders, would require reducing service standards (which would harm those in need of the service), or slashing costs—which would entail cutting workers' wages and benefits, as well as replacing more highly-trained workers with less-qualified ones. If such cost-cutting measures were not implemented, municipalities' fear of soaring costs would most likely come true.[102]

Public funding of ambulance services in Ontario, like provincial health spending in general, stagnated until 1999. The *Expenditure Estimates* for 1999-2000 and 2000-2001 promise a rise in spending (see Table 11). This is welcome news indeed after years of stagnation. However, critics of the downloading decision are concerned that ambulance services could still lose out to tax cuts or other spending priorities in the lean world of municipal budget-making.

As of March 2000:
- The downloading of ambulance services had gone through in four regional municipalities (Durham, Niagara, York, and Haldimand-

Table 11 Provincial government expenditures on ambulances, 1994-2001						
Year	Expenditures in current $	Health care price index (2000=100)	Expenditures in 2000 $	Population of Ontario	Per capita expenditures in 2000 $
1994-1995	$211,848,168	91.2	$232,289,658	10,828,000	$21.45
1995-1996	$213,625,278	92.5	$230,946,246	10,965,000	$21.06
1996-1997	$218,752,151	93.9	$232,962,887	11,101,000	$20.99
1997-1998	$228,698,760	95.6	$239,224,644	11,260,000	$21.25
1998-1999	$214,326,372	98.9	$216,710,184	11,412,000	$18.99
1999-2000 (est)	$283,606,000	100.0	$283,606,000	11,549,000	$24.56
2000-2001 (est)	$322,741,800	103.0	$313,341,553	11,699,000	$26.78

Source: Public Accounts of Ontario, 1995-1999, and Expenditure Estimates, 1999-2001; Statistics Canada, CANSIM Matrix P106085 (inflation projected at 3% in 2000-2001); Canadian Institute for Health Information (population growth projected at 1.298% 2000-2001 forward); Bill Murnighan, "Health Care Spending in Ontario." Ontario Alternative Budget Working Group, Paper No. 8, April 2000.

Norfolk). In two cases, the county had begun operating a region-wide service, in one a hospital had taken over such a service, and in the fourth the county had renewed the contracts of the existing providers.
- Six further regional municipalities (Haliburton, Halton, Hamilton-Wentworth, Huron, Lambton, and Ottawa-Carleton) had decided to provide ambulance services in-house.
- Six others (Lanark, Middlesex, Muskoka, Oxford, Peel, and Victoria) had selected outside service providers. Two had opted for a hospital-based service, two were negotiating with existing providers, one had chosen a new, commercial provider, while one was negotiating with new and existing providers.
- Four municipalities had issued RFPs (Bruce, Chatham-Kent, Grey, and Simcoe).
- Eleven other municipalities had not yet selected a delivery model or service providers (Brant, Essex, Frontenac, Hastings, Lennox-Addington, Prince Edward, Renfrew; Leeds-Grenville, Nipissing, Northumberland, Parry Sound, Prescott-Russell, Stormont, Dundas & Glengarry, Sudbury, and Wellington.[104]

In March 2000, about half of the upper-tier municipalities had already decided on a model and providers. Of these sixteen, eight (50 percent) had decided to provide the service themselves; three (20 percent) had opted for hospital-based services; four (25 percent) had opted for the existing providers or are negotiating with them; and one (5 percent) had chosen a commercial provider. It is too soon to tell what will become of Ontario's ambulance services. What the remaining fifteen municipalities choose to do will be crucial.[105]

User charges and de-insured services

Conservative Health Minister Jim Wilson and Premier Mike Harris both declared after the 1995 election that their government would not introduce any new user fees for services covered by the Canada Health Act—leaving the door open to user fees for services not covered by the Act.[106] And indeed, at their August 1995 conference, the provincial premiers asked Ottawa to allow "greater flexibility in the design and delivery" of health care and other social programs. They called for the creation of a "commonly accepted definition" of medical services "essential to the health and well-being of Canadians." These would be covered by medicare. Other services would or could be de-listed and subject to user fees. Speaking to journalists, Premier Harris said that user fees might be necessary. Pointing to de-listing of services under the NDP and co-payments under the Liberals, he said "You've got to realize that de-listing something is a 100 per cent user fee for what somebody considers necessary."[107]

By September 1995, the *Ottawa Citizen* was announcing the government's intention to make seniors pay more for drugs, in order to reduce expenditures under the Ontario Drug Benefit plan, breaking the promise made in the Common Sense Revolution election platform.[108] Under the Ontario Drug Benefit plan, all senior citizens and people living on social assistance received free prescription drugs. With Bill 26, the Harris government introduced a $2 "co-payment" per prescription for social assistance recipients and seniors receiving the Guaranteed Income Supplement. In addition, beneficiaries of the ODB earning individual incomes over $16,140 per year, or family incomes over $24,000 per year, were faced with paying a $100 annual deductible and the pharmacists' dispensing fees (up to $6.11 per prescription). In 1997-1998, the total cost of the government's drug benefit plans was $1.3 billion, but recipients accounted for $200 million of that directly in "co-payments." In 1998-1999, the total cost was $1.4 billion, while recipients had to pay $215 million.[109] Senior citizens and social assistance recipients are thus paying about 15 percent of the cost directly.

Health economist Robert Evans has referred to medical user fees as "zombies": " ideas that are intellectually dead but will not stay in their graves."[110] Allegedly introduced to restore equity and fiscal balance, their impact is entirely negative. The user charges for drugs have the effect of weakening a program brought in specifically to assist the members of the community who bear by far the greatest burden of drug costs, namely the elderly, and those who are least able financially to bear the cost, namely the poorest citizens, who depend on social assistance. By shifting part of the cost back from healthier and wealthier citizens to unhealthier and "unwealthier" ones, the user charges for prescription drugs run counter to the guiding principle of medicare, and are regressive.

Bill 26 authorized hospitals to charge a fee of $26.94 per day to patients in acute-care hospitals who "refused" to move to a chronic-care facility. The fee would be deemed to cover "room and board" and would match what a patient would pay in a chronic care hospital or nursing home. Under the Canada Health Act, no medically necessary service can be billed directly to a patient. Ontario Ministry of Health spokesperson Paul Kilbertus "said the plan is only to charge it to people who refuse to move from a general hospital to a chronic-care facility because they don't want to pay for room and board."[111] As of January 1, 1997, the fee was raised to $40.29 a day, the amount charged to people in nursing homes, homes for the aged and other long-term care institutions. A 60-day waiting period was also dropped, enabling hospitals to impose the fee "as soon as a doctor has certified that a patient is 'more or less permanently' living in the hospital." It was estimated that 20 per cent of the beds in Ontario's general hospitals were occupied by patients waiting for a spot in a nursing home—some 5,000 people.[112] The co-payment was increased every year; effective July 1, 2000, it went up to $43.03 per day, or $1,308.89 per month.[113] These fees represent a terrible financial burden, especially considering the fact that 49 percent of unattached women aged 65 or older live in poverty.[114]

The Ministry of Health and Ontario Medical Association reviewed the OHIP benefit schedule in 1997 "with a view to removing outmoded or cosmetic procedures, and achieving better value for health spending."[115] Following on the review, OHIP delisted twenty-two services deemed obsolete or marginal. These included eight cosmetic procedures, including certain kinds of wart removal, procedures to remove acne-blemished skin, "insertion of a prosthesis to replace a surgically removed testicle," and male mastectomy to counter "non-diseased overdevelopment of the breast."[116] At the same time, it "redefined" standards of care for some services and "clarified" physicians' billing practices. The Ministry of Health declared that the changes would save $50 million.[117]

In addition, the government declared that the Ontario Health Insurance Plan would henceforth pay for eye examinations only every two years for most people between 20 and 64.[118] Flu vaccinations would be funded only for high risk patients.

As of July 1998, the Ministry of Health ceased paying any part of the cost of "pre-departure travel medicine services that travellers obtain solely for the purpose of travel outside Canada [including] assessments, counselling or the administration of vaccines or drugs for prevention of communicable diseases no endemic to Canada." From October 1, 1998 on, it deleted gender re-assignment surgery from the list of insured services.[119]

Primary care

Bill 26 aroused considerable vocal opposition among physicians, as it challenged their power and freedom to do business. The power struggle between physicians and the state is not a new phenomenon. The medical profession was throughout the 20th century at the apex of the division of labour in health care; it "had the power to exclude, limit or subordinate other health occupations." However, recent years have seen this power challenged and constrained by governments seeking to rationalize health care in order to control its cost and its development, as well as by other health care professions striving for greater autonomy and powers of self-regulation.[120] On the one hand, governments enacted legislation enhancing the autonomy of those other professions, such as midwives or nurse practitioners (see below). On the other hand, they moved to wrest control of the cost of physicians' services from the medical profession itself. When public insurance for physicians' services was introduced in Ontario in 1971, the Ontario Medical Association (OMA) established the schedule of fees. By the late 1970s, the provincial government began to set fees itself under the Ontario Health Insurance Plan (OHIP) in negotiation with the OMA. Many physicians reacted to the discrepancy between the fees set by OHIP and the higher ones proposed by the OMA by billing patients for the difference. This practice of "extra-billing" was outlawed by the federal government in the 1984 *Canada Health Act*. Yet physicians were still able to raise the amount they billed OHIP by increasing the volume of services they performed (by accepting more patients, etc.). The provincial government then introduced other cost-containment measures. It promoted community health centres, in which physicians are on salary. It also took steps to limit the overall number of physicians and cap the global amount physicians as a whole can bill OHIP.[121] In 1991, the NDP government negotiated a framework agreement with the OMA, under which a soft cap was placed on OHIP's funding pool—i.e. if total medical expenditures exceeded a predefined limit, fees paid to individual physicians would be clawed back. Individual physicians would also only receive a percentage of all amounts billed beyond $400,000.[122]

According to David Coburn, there was at first little sympathy between the Conservative government and the medical profession: "There was neither a congruence of interests nor much social interaction between medicine and a highly ideological market-oriented government. To the New Right, health care is simply another area requiring rationalization, the discipline of the market, and more competition. Physicians were viewed as highly paid monopolists."[123] At first, the Harris government maintained the hard line heralded in Bill 26, proposing in 1996 a 10 per cent clawback for billings under $251,000, 33 per cent for billings between $251,000 and $276,000, 67 per cent for billings between $276,000 and $301,000, and 75 per cent for any billings above $301,000. A year-long dispute with physicians ensued, culminating in a five-week strike by some specialists in the fall of 1996. While a settlement was reached, Health Minister Jim Wilson stated in December 1996 that new user fees might have to be introduced to pay for its estimated $300 million annual cost.[124]

In fact, it can hardly be claimed that the province's transfer payments to physicians and other primary care practitioners went through the roof. As Table 12 shows, per capita provincial spending on such services and care dropped in real terms after 1995. Even in 2000-2001, at a time when overall health spending has increased, per capita expenditures on primary care practitioners and physicians will only be $491.93 (in constant 2000 dollars), whereas they were $500.90 in 1994-1995.

In the midst of the dispute with the physicians, Health Minister Jim Wilson announced that the government would "soon introduce legislation to recognize and strengthen the role of the nurse practitioner in primary care," carrying to fruition a project initiated by the previous, NDP, government. The passage of this legislation, Bill 127, provides a useful example of the intersection of a holistic, social model of community health care with a managerial model of cost containment. On the one hand, nurse practitioners bring to medical practice a different perspective than physicians. Their orientation is very much to holistic medicine and health promotion. Introducing more nurse-practitioners into the health care system therefore appeals to an ideology of community health intent on breaking down the barriers between health care and social services. At the same time, nurse practitioners can offer some of the same services as physicians[125], but at a much lower cost (in terms of education, salary, etc.).[126] Nurse-practitioners therefore also seem very attractive from a cost-containment point of view.

Table 12
Transfer payments made for services and care provided by physicians and other practitioners, 1995-2001

Year	Total spending (current $)	Health care price index (2000=100)	Total spending (2000 $)	Population of Ontario	Per capita spending (2000 $)
1994-1995	$4,947,141,198	91.2	$5,424,496,928	10,828,000	$500.97
1995-1996	$4,703,606,534	92.5	$5,084,980,037	10,965,000	$463.75
1996-1997	$4,863,070,597	93.9	$5,178,988,921	11,101,000	$466.53
1997-1998	$5,279,011,575	95.6	$5,521,978,635	11,260,000	$490.41
1998-1999	$5,336,812,225	98.9	$5,396,170,096	11,412,000	$472.85
1999-2000 (est)	$5,529,516,100	100.0	$5,529,516,100	11,549,000	$478.79
2000-2001 (est)	$5,922,443,600	103.0	$5,749,945,243	11,690,000	$491.87

Source: Public Accounts of Ontario, 1995-1999, and Expenditure Estimates, 1999-2001, Statistics Canada, CANSIM Matrix P106085 (inflation projected at 3% in 2000-2001); Canadian Institute for Health Information (population growth projected at 1.298% 2000-2001 forward); Bill Murnighan, "Health Care Spending in Ontario," Ontario Alternative Budget Working Group, Paper No. 8, April 2000.

The cost-containment perspective has been especially influential in the debate about nurse practitioners in Ontario: "The arguments for cost-effectiveness were particularly attractive to provincial governments across Canada which were trying to control health-care costs, and this became evident in report after report by government appointed committees."[127] The holistic, community health discourse has provided a progressive veneer to the discussion, but has not been the determining factor. The emphasis has been on the *curative* model of health care and on the relative cost of physicians and nurse-practitioners, rather than on the broader caring function and the benefits to patients of more holistic medicine.[128]

Although the initiative to establish nurse practitioners as a new class of health care professionals had long been discussed, it appears that Ruth Grier's appointment as Health Minister in the NDP government led to action finally being taken. However, there were many delays and legislation was not proclaimed until 1998, under the Conservative government. This continuity can be explained by both governments' central concern with cost-containment. Health Minister Jim Wilson announced in December 1996 that he would "soon introduce legislation to recognize and strengthen the role of the nurse practitioner in primary care." The timing was interesting—during a five-week-long protest action by many of Ontario's physicians. This may suggest "that the Conservative government's continued support of nurse practitioners was related to its negotiations with the medical profession."[129]

Under the Health Insurance Act, a physician may bill a patient for a service that is not publicly insured. During their dispute with the government, physicians in a number of Ontario towns announced that they would immediately begin to bill patients directly for services which they did not charge to OHIP, such as notes to employers on behalf of sick employees, information for Workers' Compensation, or transferring files. The physicians declared that they would either bill patients per service rendered or would charge them an annual fee. The range reportedly approved by physicians in London, for example, was $150 to $175 a year for a family with two children or more, $90 to $100 for a person over 18 and $45 to $60 for a person under 18 years.[130] Some physicians were also reportedly asking patients for "tips" as a way of getting back the 10 percent clawback imposed by the government. In September 1998, the Medical Reform Group charged that some physicians were resorting to "creative extra-billing" in contravention of the Canada Health Act.[131]

In June 1995, the Ontario Divisional Court had struck down a government regulation forbidding physicians from charging annual fees for transferring records, filling out forms and doing consultations over the phone. Between 1987 and 1993, physicians had been allowed to charge such annual fees. In 1993, NDP Health Minister Ruth Grier had ordered the College of Physicians and Surgeons to pass a regulation against this. Patients had then been billed for each individual service not covered by OHIP. For example, "at one Bloor St. W. medical practice, patients were charged $30 for telephone advice during office hours, $15 for repeat prescriptions and $25 for every 15 minutes of travelling to the patient's home."[132]

Meanwhile, Dr. Bill Orovan, head of the OMA, declared that increased physicians' billings were mainly due to a growing and aging population. However, he said that the OMA was also looking into *patients'* abuse of the system, and had set up a committee to document it and recommend a strategy for dealing with it. "If there is documented abuse, the committee is mandated to take action."[133] The government and medical establishment have persistently raised the spectre of patient abuse, although evidence of it is merely anecdotal.[134] Indeed, health economists have established that demand for health care is producer-driven, not the result of willful over-consumption by patients.

With a view to restructuring primary care in order to contain costs in the longer term, in June 1996 the government announced a reform plan based on the rostering of patients and the replacement of fee-for-service by capitation payments. This plan called for each patient to be assigned to a physician's roster. A patient could choose the physician, but would then have to receive all primary care from that physician once the choice was made. Patients would have to give notice they wanted to change physicians several months ahead of time. Those seeking care from another physician without giving such notice would have to pay their medical bills themselves. Physicians' rosters would be assessed by the government, which would fund their practices on a scale varying according to patients' age and gender. In exchange for being rostered, patients would receive additional services from their physician: round-the-clock medical advice over a toll-free telephone line; access to Ontario Drug Benefit plan data; one-stop access to the entire health-care system.[135] Ideas such as this had been part of public debate for some time and a number of blueprints had been proposed.[136]

Although Health Minister Jim Wilson announced in June 1996 that pilot projects would be set up to test the new model, it was not until March 1998 that the OMA board of directors approved them. Jim Wilson's successor, Elizabeth Witmer, did not announce the location of the pilot projects until May 1998.[137] Under the revised model, groups of physicians would come together (in an integrated network, although not necessarily in one physical location) to share a roster of patients. Offering a range of specializations, they could also work with nurse practitioners and midwives. Physicians would be paid on a fee-for-service basis, but would also receive bonuses for practicing preventative medicine. The government had by this time dropped the idea of charging user fees to patients seeking medical help outside of their assigned clinic, because it had been deemed contrary to the Canada Health Act.[138]

In May 2000, the Ministry of Health and the Ontario Medical Association (OMA) reached a tentative agreement in negotiating a new compensation package for the province's physicians. The four-year deal, ratified by the OMA's members, increases fee-for-service payments by 1.95 percent in the first year and 2 percent in each of the three following years. Billing thresholds will continue to apply, but at new levels which have not yet been announced. Furthermore, the province will introduce a series of new fees and incentives to encourage physicians to be more available to their patients (incentives to general practitioners to continue providing obstetrical services; incentives to ensure the availability of on-call services; incentives to physicians required to make services available around the clock; a Complex Care Premium that would recognize the additional time required to address the needs of the frail elderly; incentives to provide faster admission to emergency departments). The deal also includes new maternity leave provisions for physicians, as well as the recommendation from the Ministry of Health that the government allow physicians to incorporate their practices.

Community health centres (CHCs) have for many years provided an alternative to fee-for-service medicine and are widely recognized as a model of non-profit, integrated primary health care. The new plan would seem to chart a diametrically opposed course. Some commentators have raised the concern that it could be a vehicle for further development of a corporate form of health care:

> These new clinics are very similar to the Managed Care clinics now operating in the United States. The majority there are for-profit operations, and the establishment of similar clinics here may make it easier for private, for-profit operators of U.S. or Canadian nationality to move in. This has already happened with walk-in clinics (which, unlike CHCs and the new pilot project clinics, are not based on providing on-going service to a stable popula-

tion) and with a newly developed doctors' house-call business in Ontario.[139]

Inasmuch as the new model moves away from fee-for-service and integrates individual physicians more and more into health-service networks and managed care settings, it represents a further departure from the model of the physician as an autonomous professional towards a situation in which the physician is more tightly controlled by the state and, potentially, private corporate interests, notably in the insurance industry. Unlike the CHCs, this model is also strictly medical; it does not create a network of health and *social* services.

Finally, the Ontario Health Coalition has accused the government of wanting to pay for the new deal by de-listing a further $50 million worth of services from OHIP. As evidence for this, the Coalition points to clause 13.1 of the government's agreement with the Ontario Medical Association, which says: "The parties agree that by December 31, 2000, they shall identify changes in the existing Schedule of Benefits which will result in annual savings of at least $50 million. This will be accomplished by a mix of tightening and modernization. The process for identifying and making the changes will be agreed upon by the parties."[140]

Conclusion

Despite its protestations to the contrary, the Ontario government in fact reduced spending on health care in real per capita terms over the second half of the 1990s. The Institutional Health and Health Insurance programs together account for two-thirds of provincial health expenditures and they were hard hit. The Harris government followed its predecessors in squeezing hospital budgets and capping billing by physicians and private laboratories. Other areas were also affected by cuts, however, particularly because of the cascading impact of restructuring and privatization. The government gave itself great powers to override the decisions of local authorities and boards, while downloading services to them without their consent. Individual citizens had to pay more out-of-pocket for health care, particularly the most vulnerable who were faced with new user charges. And—although no dollar figure can be placed on this—the burden of unpaid care work increased. Faced with budget cuts, institutions such as hospitals moved further down the road to commercialization, adopting private-sector management strategies, contracting work out to the corporate sector, entering into public-private partnerships. The government moved ahead with a model of primary care reform which could encourage the development of new private clinics, offering new openings for the corporate sector. Overall, the balance tipped from the public towards the private sector. Finally, Ontario has laid the groundwork for public hospitals to have greater recourse to charity (both by providing incentives for increased charitable donations to hospitals and by in effect privatizing some of the decisions on how to spend public monies). In the final analysis, individuals and families are experiencing the impact of all the cuts and restructuring in the form of higher costs, lower levels of care, or greater anxiety about their health.

The effects of these trends are literally hitting home. *Home* is where the dollars are supposed to be flowing in the form of long-term community health services—home care. The latter has been presented as the great hope for the future of health care throughout the industrialized world. Its promise: to offer a cheaper, but more effective, alternative to institutional care in all its forms. Is the picture any different there, or does home care display the same tendencies as the rest of the health care system? This is the subject of the next chapter.

Chapter 3
Home Care

"It is easy to reduce public expenditure on a service by transferring the costs to users and carers. But this does not reduce costs, it merely redistributes them. The transfer of a public service to outside contractors may appear to produce savings, but this may not lead to greater efficiency if the savings are made at the expense of lower standards of service and poorer pay and conditions of work for employees. The lowest bid in a system of competitive tendering may not be the best option."

"There are also problems of measuring output and agreeing on appropriate criteria for appraising services. What is the output of a home providing residential care for elderly people? There is always the danger that only the measurable will be taken into account. In a residential home, for example, the physical facilities are quantifiable, but they are less important than the quality of the human relationships that characterize the home."[1]

Introduction

Home care arouses enormous interest nowadays. Although health-care experts have talked about it for years as a key link in an integrated, community-based health-care system, it has gained considerable prominence both in the discourse of politicians and in the media. In the last general election, the federal Liberal Party included a national home care program in its list of promises. As discussed in the previous chapter, there is a tendency to justify certain health-care expenditures or innovations (such as an increased role for nurse-practitioners) by invoking the holistic, integrated community health services paradigm, while in fact opting for them out of essentially financial reasons. Home care appears to fall into this category as well.

This chapter will tell some of the story of home care in Ontario over the past five years,

- as the province opted for managed competition in home care, a market-based system of allocating funds and choosing service providers;
- as the province put money into agencies, yet those agencies could not meet the public demand for services;
- as venerable, highly respected home care providers closed down and new ones sprang up, and the for-profit sector gained new footholds in the sector.

The overall conclusion of the analysis is that the balance has been tipping in the home care sector as it has elsewhere in the health-care system:

- patients and dollars are being moved out of the institutions insured under the Canada Health Act (hospitals) into those which are not (long-term care or home care), with the resulting loss of standards (universality, accessibility, portability, comprehensiveness, and public administration);
- home care services have increased, yet they are rationed and people in need must purchase much of the care they need privately and especially rely on the unpaid labour of family and friends;
- the administration and delivery of home care services is more and more governed by the logic of profit and competition;
- the allocation of home care dollars is shrouded in secrecy as a result of privatization.

The chapter is divided into five sections, each of which is itself divided into smaller parts:

a) Why care and costs are being shifted into the community sector
b) Home care is rationed
c) Re-engineering home care: the introduction of managed competition
d) The impact of managed competition
e) Conclusion

The analysis draws on data provided by the Ontario Ministry of Health and Long-Term Care, as well as on published reports and documents. It is also based on interviews I conducted between August 1999 and April 2000, as well as on two surveys of Community Care Access Centres (CCACs) I conducted in August/September 1999 and in December 1999/January 2000. In both cases, questionnaires were mailed to all CCACs. In the first survey, I subsequently went over the answers to the questionnaire with CEOs or senior managers of most of the CCACs. In the second survey, CCACs were contacted by telephone to solicit participation, but personal interviews did not take place. The response rate to the first questionnaire was 67 percent, to the second 58 percent. The second survey was supplemented by a telephone and fax mini-survey in April 2000.

Many people associated with CCACs and provider agencies gave very generously of their time and knowledge. They are intelligent, caring, dedicated and open-minded individuals with much experience and expertise. I should like to stress that the criticisms voiced in this chapter are in no way intended to reflect on the work or abilities of the individuals who work in the sector and are putting much effort into improving the lives of their fellow citizens.

Defining home care

The Federal/Provincial/Territorial Working Group on Home Care (1990) defined it as "an array of services which enables clients incapacitated in whole or in part to live at home, often with the effect of preventing, delaying or substituting for long-term care or acute care alternatives."[2] Home care comprises two streams: professional services, such as nursing, occupational therapy and physiotherapy; and home support services, such as homemaking, personal care, housekeeping, and transportation. In addition, home care may include adult day programs, meal programs, home maintenance, respite care, medical equipment and supplies, and counselling.[3] These are laid out in Ontario's *Long-Term Care Act, 1994*, which defines community services as community support services, homemaking services, personal support services and professional services. These in turn are defined as follows:

- *Community support services*: "meal services, transportation services, caregiver support services, adult day programs, home maintenance and repair services, friendly visiting services, security checks or reassurance services, social or recreational services, providing prescribed equipment, supplies or other goods, services prescribed as community support services" (where "'prescribed' means prescribed by the regulations").
- *Homemaking services*: "housecleaning, doing laundry, ironing, mending, shopping, banking, paying bills, planning menus, preparing meals, caring for children, assisting a person with any of [these activities], training a person to carry out or assist with any of [these activities], providing prescribed equipment, supplies or other goods, services prescribed as homemaking services."
- *Personal support services*: "personal hygiene activities, routine personal activities of living, assisting a person with any of [these activi-

ties], training a person to carry out or assist with any of [these activities], providing prescribed equipment, supplies or other goods, services prescribed as personal support services."
- *Professional services*: "nursing services, occupational therapy services, physiotherapy services, social work services, speech-language pathology services, dietetics services, training a person to provide any of [these services], providing prescribed equipment, supplies or other goods, services prescribed as professional services."[4]

Why care and costs are being shifted into the community sector

The push to move more and more care from institutions into the community seeks a justification in a progressive vision of health and social services, as we have seen in earlier chapters. Progressive health-care reformers have long believed that everything must be done to enable those in need of care to receive it safely and independently in their homes if possible, rather than in acute-care hospitals or other institutions. But they have also stressed that this can be a reasonable option only if it is medically and socially appropriate, and if the necessary infrastructure and resources are in place. But as we have seen, governments have not waited to create those infrastructures; they have cut, restructured, downloaded, and imposed user charges. It is more likely that the *real driving force of the shift to home care has been governments' desire to reduce costs*.

There are two main ways of reducing costs: making it cheaper to provide services and not providing them at all.
- Wages are the major cost in human services and that is where governments have looked for savings in making services cheaper to produce.
- The major source of home care is the informal work of unpaid care givers. Governments have downloaded service provision and costs onto them by removing care from the hospitals where it is publicly insured to the home, where it is not; this has allowed them to ration care. This is a classic example of *cascading privatization*: a shift from the insured to the uninsured zone (hospital to home) leads to the replacement of public sector by private providers, both for-profit and informal.

Governments want to cut wage costs

As a leading authority on home care points out, there are several reasons for the growth in interest in home care, but certainly *"a key motivating factor appears to be the common belief that significant public sector cost-savings may be realized by redirecting care away from institutions towards the community."*[5] For governments concerned with rising spending, home care is widely thought to offer a very attractive alternative to care in a hospital.[6]

Whether it really does save money or not is a matter of some controversy. University of Toronto researchers who examined the issue for the Institute of Clinical Evaluative Sciences state that a "disturbing aspect of the growth in home care spending has been the lack of compelling evidence that home care services are a cost-effective alternative for institutional care." They further suggest that, "in the absence of evidence-based decision making, health system restructuring may result in more, not less, costly patterns of practice, and erode, not enhance, health outcomes."[7] On the other hand, a study conducted in Saskatchewan, "looked at whether home care could effectively, safely, and at reduced costs, be provided as a substitute for non-acute hospital care." It concluded "that, while health outcomes are the same, it costs $850 more overall to care for recovering patients in hospital than it does to discharge them and provide follow-up home care."[8]

Most recently, the National Evaluation of the Cost-Effectiveness of Home Care, sponsored by the federal government's Health Transition Fund, concluded that the average "overall health care costs to government for clients in home care range from one half to three quarters of the costs for clients in facility care."[9] The savings could be as high as fifty percent of the total cost, *"provided elderly clients were stable in their type and level of care."*[10] This is a crucial *if*—the researchers found that the savings vanished the sicker the patient got. Indeed: "For clients who died the costs were higher in home care. (...) when clients go into long-term care institutions, their facility costs increase but their use of other services decreases. (...) staff at residential facilities may be able to care for client needs so that they do not need to be admitted to acute care hospitals as often."[11]

There is another big question mark here, though: research director Marcus Hollander "stressed that it is not yet known *whether the burden of costs is simply shifted onto the shoulders of clients and their caregivers."*[12] And that, no doubt, is the nub of the question. As we saw in Chapter 2, *the key strategies of cost containment involve lowering wage costs by replacing higher paid by lower paid workers, and by replacing paid workers by workers who are not paid at all—family, neighbours, friends, volunteers.* When all is said and done, *labour costs less in the home care sector.*

Workers in the home care sector are underpaid

The largely unregulated home care workforce in Canada comprised some 75,000 visiting homemakers and some 55,000 nurses in 1996. The majority of visiting homemakers are female part-time employees "receiving few fringe benefits, and with few career options within the field"—a field that pays some of the lowest wages, even in comparison with other occupations deemed to require low skill levels, notably in other health-care sectors, such as hospitals and long-term-care facilities ("average earnings for full-time year-round workers were $26,900 in 1995, well below the average of $35,700 for all occupations"[13]). The Nursing Task Force appointed by the Ontario government found that registered nurses working in home care made $16 to $23 an hour, while their counterparts in hospitals earned $19 to $28 an hour. The Ontario Community Support Association, which represents non-profit agencies, notes that personal-support workers make $5 to $8 an hour less in the community sector than in long-term-care facilities. It has called for elimination of this disparity as a condition of stability in home care.[14] The Ontario Home Health Care Providers' Association (OHHCPA), which represents for-profit agencies, echoes this, pointing out that entry-level wages for personal-support workers are $3 to $5 an hour higher in long-term-care facilities; for nurses, the gap is $4 to $8 an hour. The OHHCPA recommends "that the community care sector must be resourced adequately so that wages can rise in home care. Wage rates across all sectors of health care must narrow, so that shortages of staff do not occur in one sector at the expense of another sector." It also recommends "that compensation packages in the home-care sector need to include appropriate market wages and benefits including: short-term disability, long-term disability, permanency of hours, pension, health and dental benefits or percentage in lieu of benefits, reimbursement for mileage and travel time."[15]

Home care workers' weekly work schedules are often uncertain. Split shifts and staggered work weeks are common occurrences for them. Their prospects for career advancement in the field are scant. There is, not surprisingly, high staff turnover in home care. Yet, given mounting demand for and spending on services, home care is ironically the fourth fastest growing among 139 listed job categories.[16]

Informal caregivers bear most of the burden

Informal care givers provide 75 to 85 percent of the help that seniors receive in the community.[17] Half of those care givers experience the repercussions of this in their jobs (days of employment lost, etc.), while 40 percent must cope with additional out-of-pocket expenditures.

Reporting on interviews with 1,500 working Canadians, a study by the Conference Board of Canada points out that one quarter of Canadian workers provide care or support of some kind to an elderly friend or relative, with one quarter of those individuals providing personal care (feeding, dressing, bathing). The percentage of workers in the "sandwich generation" (those who look after both elderly people and children) has increased from 9.5 to 15 per cent. The increasing burden of work itself leads to increased health care costs, because of its detrimental impact on care givers' health.[18] A survey conducted for We Care Health Services, a home care provider agency, found that family caregivers suffer from burnout, a sense of helplessness, isolation and financial hardship. Over 90 percent reported experiencing sleep deprivation, anxiety, guilt and isolation, 70 percent reported depression, and over 60 percent reported deteriorating health.[19]

Home care is rationed

Finally, it must be remembered that home care is not covered by medicare as physician and hospital care are. Hospitals are insured services under the Canada Health Act. They cannot turn away a patient who has been admitted by a physician. Home care agencies, by contrast, offer "extended health services,"[20] and do not have the same obligation to provide care. The Toronto Community Care Access Centre, which brokers home care services in Toronto on behalf of the Ministry of Health and Long-Term Care, says that this has opened the door to privatization:

> In Ontario the swing to shorter hospital stays and an expanding list of medical procedures performed as day surgery or on an outpatient basis means that a large portion of treatment and recovery is now done outside the hospital environment in private homes, shelters, or long-term care facilities. This has led to a gradual shift toward privatization. While public insurance covers all costs of treatment and recovery during a hospital stay, once the care moves beyond the hospital walls patients are no longer fully insured. The province covers some costs, but the individual

may be charged for nursing, medication, homemaking, or medical equipment or supplies. And the insured services vary from province to province with Ontario offering the most widespread coverage. Because the Canada Health Act does not encompass home care, the federal government has no specific ground on which to oppose this trend away from the founding tenets of medicare. Coverage is no longer either universal or portable as each province goes its own way. Accessibility is now dependent on such factors as waiting lists, and affordability has also been compromised by the mounting number of services charged directly to patients. Public administration may well stand as the one criteria (sic) that remains intact. Medicare is now subject to the vagaries of changing governments and variations in policies. And the impact is felt most strongly in the areas of convalescent care and social support services provided in the home and in the community.[21]

Home care services are rationed. In 1999, the Ontario government introduced regulations to the 1994 Long-Term Care Act defining eligibility for homemaking services and the maximum amount of nursing, homemaking, and personal support services for which a person is eligible.[22]

Regulation 2 (1) states that a CCAC shall deem a person eligible to receive homemaking services if:
- "the person requires personal support services along with the homemaking services;
- "the person receives personal support and homemaking services from a caregiver who requires assistance with the homemaking services in order to continue providing the person with all the required care;
- "the person requires constant supervision as a result of a cognitive impairment or acquired brain injury and the person's caregiver requires assistance with the homemaking services."[23]

The regulation goes on to cap the amount of nursing, homemaking and personal support services a person may receive. With respect to homemaking and personal support services, it stipulates that CCACs shall not provide a person with more than "80 hours, in the first 30 days that follow the first day of service" and "60 hours, in any subsequent 30-day period." However, a CCAC may provide more hours of service for a maximum of 30 days if it "determines that there exists (sic) extraordinary circumstances that justify the provision of additional services." In the case of nursing, the ceiling is "the lesser" of:

1. "28 visits from a registered nurse or a registered practical nurse in a seven-day period;
2. "The following number of hours of service in a seven-day period:
i "If services are provided by registered nurses, 43 hours of service,
ii "If services are provided by registered practical nurses, 53 hours of service, or
iii "If the services are provided by both registered nurses and registered practical nurses, 48 hours of service."[24]

These regulations are said to regularize and standardize what had already been the general practice across the province.[25]

These regulations call for two comments. First, the nature of the population receiving home care visits is changing. With an increasing proportion of home care recipients seriously ill or recovering from surgery, and with an increasing proportion of frail elderly clients, the number and length of visits needed in the past may no longer suffice. What is notable about these regulations as well, is that they are entirely concerned with establishing *eligibility and its limits*, not with defining *rights*. In this sense, they appear to be essentially another cost-containing measure.

Secondly, it does not appear to be the case that they simply formalize a universal practice. On the contrary, there seem to be at least some places where home care was regarded as an entitlement, as a service to be provided to those in need, not as a scarce commodity to be rationed. For example, a "Backgrounder" produced by the Kingston, Frontenac, Lennox & Addington Community Care Access Centre states:

> Home care in Canada is an anomaly in the health-care system. Unlike hospital care, home care does not fall under the federal Canada Health Act. If it did, people would be entitled to home care (which they are not), just as they are entitled to hospital care. Until 1995 in Ontario, however, home care was interpreted to be an entitlement program under the Health Insurance Act and the Homemaking and Nurses Services Act. Ontario residents could therefore receive home-nursing and homemaking services when they needed them. When the home-care program overspent its budget because of increased demand for services, the provincial government supplemented the home-care budget. But new policies, which were introduced by the former New Democratic government and maintained by the current Progressive Conservative Government, eliminated this entitlement. Today, if the need for services is greater than an Access Centre's annual budget, the Centre may have to allocate services to those with the greatest

need. This year, the local Access Centre had waiting lists for many services, and it has developed policies and guidelines to help care managers decide who needs services the most. The Centre is committed to providing the best service available with its limited funding."[26]

Finally, one has to ask what rationing guidelines are not written into the Regulations per se, but exist just the same. For example, in a draft document sent to Community Care Access Centres and other long-term care community agencies in 1999, the Ministry of Health and Long-Term Care proposed not just a methodology for setting maximum service levels, but also eligibility criteria for various services, and guidelines for giving priority to some service users over others.[27] One of the criteria to be used to determine whether a person was eligible to receive long-term care community services was: "Caregiving or support required by the person exceeds the ability of the person's relatives, friends and the capability of other community resources." Although the definition of this criterion in the document is surrounded by qualifying statements stressing that the Ministry's intention is to help those who are looking after their friends or relatives, it is hard to get around the fact that this implicitly says that friends and relatives are the main source of eldercare, *not by default, because the resources are not there, but because it ought to be so.*

Again, the document proposes guidelines for giving some people priority access to services over others. There are two categories: (a) those at risk of dying or in need of care within 24 hours; and (b) those whose health would be compromised or who would have to be institutionalized if care were not forthcoming in a timely fashion. The guidelines state that those in the first category must be served before those in the second. While it is common sense to suggest that those in greater danger should receive attention first, the implication of this guideline is that the services are not and cannot be available for everyone—if they were, there would be no need for such a guideline.

This document illustrates how inadequate funding of home care is translated not just into a lack of services, but into a particular outlook and set of practices. The limits of the public sector are tightly circumscribed here as rationing becomes encoded in lasting norms and guidelines.

In conclusion, then, the push to move care from institutions into the home can *in the abstract* be justified as better for many patients. But the driving force today is the government's policy of cutting costs, at the expense of paid workers (because of diminished compensation), unpaid workers (because of extra work, expenses and stress), and of patients and users (because care is rationed and no longer fully insured), especially women with lower incomes. In this context, the superior advantages of home care are at least questionable.

Funding has increased, but does it suffice?

And yet, has government spending on home care not increased? Indeed, home care has received a growing share of public health care spending over the past twenty years, going from about one percent of the total in 1980 to over five percent in 2000. The 1980s in particular saw spectacular annual increases averaging over twenty-five percent. In 1980, Ontario spent $46 million on home care, in 1990 $389 million, and in 2000 $1,481 million.[28] Yet, as one provider agency executive put it: "We had a hospital-laden health care system, with just pennies put into home care. Spending may have gone up, but 200 or 300, or 500 percent of a penny is still not very much."[29]

Evidence of the rapid rise in demand can be found by looking both at the number of clients CCACs have served, and at the number of professional visits and homemaking hours they have purchased.[30] Between 1996-1997 and 1998-1999, the total number of CCAC clients increased by 20.2 percent. Only one CCAC, West Parry Sound, saw its volume of clients decline. The greatest increases were in Durham (43.5 percent) and York (42.4 percent), while the lowest were in Cochrane (1.2 percent) and Haliburton-Northumberland-Victoria (6.2 percent). An even sharper picture can be obtained by looking at the number of homemaking hours, as well as visits by nurses, physiotherapists, occupational therapists, speech-language pathologists and nutritional counsellors, provided by CCACs from 1996 to 1999. On average, nursing visits increased by 30.8 percent, homemaking hours by 24.9 percent, physiotherapy visits by 17.6 percent, occupational therapy visits by 26.7 percent (see Table 13).

Table 13
Rate of increase of average CCAC professional visits and homemaking hours, 1996-1999

	# of nursing visits	# of homemaking hours	# of physiotherapy visits	# of occupational therapy visits	# of speech-Language pathology visits	# of dietetics visits
1996-1997 Average	154,433	398,809	12,450	9,952	4,117	1,919
1997-1998 Average	178,460	468,893	13,359	11,239	4,421	2,246
% Change, 1997 to 1998	15.6	17.6	7.3	12.9	7.4	16.9
1998-1999 Average	201,953	498,248	14,645	12,609	4,947	1,586
% Change, 1998 to 1999	13.2	6.3	9.6	12.2	11.9	-29.4
% Change, 1997-1999	30.8	24.9	17.6	26.7	20.2	-17.4

Source: Based on data submitted by CCACs to the Ontario Home Care Administration System (OHCAS).

To meet the increased demand on their own resources, CCACs have been growing. In August-September 1999, 86 percent of the CCACs reported that the number of their paid employees had increased during the preceding twelve months, eleven percent reported no change, and only three percent (one CCAC) reported a decline in the number of paid staff. Seventy-six percent of CCACs expected to hire paid staff over the following twelve months, fourteen percent expected to lay off some paid staff (notably because of the provincially-imposed obligation to divest themselves of their direct-service providers, such as nurses, therapists and home-support workers), while ten percent expected neither to hire nor to lay off any paid employees. Almost all the CCACs expecting to hire staff said they would be recruiting professionals and case managers; about half also said they would be taking on additional clerical and support staff.[31]

According to the figures reported in Table 14, funding for in-home services from the Ministry of Health and Long-Term Care increased by 29.1 percent in real terms between 1996-1997 and 1998-1999. A look at the six-year period from 1994-1995 to 1999-2000 shows that 1996-1997 represents a trough, and 1997-1998 and 1998-2000 peaks, in terms of expenditure growth. Over those six years, just the same, total Ministry of Health transfer payments for home care and community services went up by 36 percent in real terms. Spending is estimated to increase by a further 2.7 percent in real terms in 2000-2001.

As Table 15 suggests, the good news is that these large spending increases roughly kept pace with the rising volume of professional vis-

Table 14
Provincial government expenditures on home care in constant (2000) dollars and per program, 1994-2001*

	Professional services	Homemaking services	Personal support/ attendant outreach	Acquired brain injury services	Supportive housing services	Children's treatment centres	Community support services	Total
1994-1995								$1,089,363,739
1995-1996	$523,678,595	$327,100,958	$27,576,638	$16,216,720	$74,138,907	$31,053,044	$116,044,676	$1,115,863,574
1996-1997	$495,341,455	$322,401,598	$27,805,155	$19,553,643	$84,424,254	$30,337,450	$117,557,516	$1,097,421,071
1997-1998	$606,990,257	$371,949,447	$35,098,129	$28,393,475	$91,871,057	$29,870,447	$110,349,702	$1,274,522,514
1998-1999	$635,292,037	$432,059,471	$39,861,077	$30,868,697	$105,243,396	$30,364,177	$142,574,995	$1,416,263,850
1999-2000 (est)	$664,142,000	$460,584,200	$33,075,400	$35,902,600	$99,262,600	$29,006,400	$159,797,800	$1,481,771,000
2000-2001 (est)	$693,048,797	$481,412,063	$32,115,875	$34,861,057	$96,846,713	$28,164,917	$155,316,998	$1,521,766,419

*In 1994-1995 program envelopes were defined differently.
Source Public Accounts of Ontario, 1995-1999, and Expenditure Estimates, 1999-2001; Statistics Canada, CANSIM Matrix P106085 (inflation projected at 3% in 2000-2001).

Table 15
Comparison of volume of homemaking hours and professional visits
with Ontario Ministry of Health funding, 1996-1999
(in constant 2000 Dollars)

	1996-1997	1997-1998		1998-1999		% Increase 1996-1999
		Service or expenditure	% Increase	Service or expenditure	% Increase	
Homemaking hours	15,154,744	17,817,938	17.6	18,933,434	6.3	24.9
Expenditures on homemaking	$322,401,598	$371,949,447	15.4	$432,059,471	16.2	34.0
Professional visits	6,992,357	8,016,001	14.6	9,056,398	13.0	29.5
Expenditures on professional visits	$495,341,455	$606,990,257	22.5	$635,292,037	4.7	28.3

Source: Based on data submitted by CCACs to the Ontario Home Care Administration System and on the *Public Accounts of Ontario, 1996-1997*.

its and homemaking hours purchased by CCACs. Between 1996-1997 and 1998-1999, the number of homemaking hours purchased by CCACs increased by 24.9 percent, while Ministry of Health transfer payments for them went up by 34.0 percent. In those same years, the number of professional visits purchased by CCACs rose by 29.5 percent, while the Ministry of Health's transfer payments for them climbed by 28.3 percent. On average, the Ministry of Health transferred $21.77 per homemaking hour in constant 1992 dollars to the CCACs in 1996-1997 and $22.82 in 1998-1999. It transferred on average $70.84 to the CCACs for professional visits in 1996-1997 and $70.15 in 1998-1999.

However, while provincial payments to the CCACs have more or less kept up with the rising volume of CCAC services, this in itself says nothing about whether either the province or the CCACs have met community needs.

Services are being cut, rationed

Sixteen out of 43 CCACs are reportedly facing a deficit in 1999-2000. Some have resorted to establishing waiting lists for services, others to trimming the amount of service offered.[32] The Toronto Community Care Access Centre reports:

> The old City of Toronto has a disproportionate number of clients who are homeless or under-housed, have mental illnesses, are HIV positive or have AIDS, are disabled or elderly and living alone: these populations are challenging to serve. Our original base funding of $55 million was insufficient to meet the needs of our clientele; in fact, we needed more than $70 million to serve our community. (…) During this period, when we were repeatedly told we must live within the allotted budget of $55 million, we were forced to drastically cut expenditures. We found our-

selves in a Catch 22 situation—we either had to reduce services or reduce the number of clients. We decided to implement changes in the criteria for some services which resulted in service cutbacks and thus cost reductions. The Board really agonized over this decision because it runs counter to our philosophy of providing support for the health, well-being and quality of life of our community. In fact, the action we had to take goes against the very core of what we believe the Toronto Community Care Access Centre stands for.[33]

Some CCACs no longer pay for as much care or equipment as they used to. For example, the Ottawa-Carleton CCAC used to pay the rent on equipment such as toilet commodes or bath benches for up to six months, but now only does so for two months. Four months' of equipment rent have been offloaded onto the client.[34] Mike Davidson, Chair of the Chatham-Kent CCAC's board of directors, told the *Chatham Daily News*: "Let's say you're entitled to five visits (for care) (...) maybe we can only give you four or three. We don't want to have a waiting list for services like other CCACs do, but maybe we have to look at that (...) We're also looking at discharging some of our cases sooner if we can." The Chatham-Kent CCAC's board has decided no longer to provide support services in rest homes, and not to increase mental health services as originally planned.[35]

The Eastern Counties CCAC in Cornwall has recently created a waiting list for services deemed a low priority, such as house-cleaning or meal preparation, because of a funding shortfall.[36] The Haldimand-Norfolk CCAC also has waiting lists. It has called on "families and individuals who use home-care services in Haldimand-Norfolk (...) to take more responsibility for their well-being." This approach is reportedly dictated by "funding constraints": "CCAC's 12-million budget (...) has remained unchanged for the past four years. Meanwhile the caseload continues to grow as the population ages." The CCAC is consequently seeking to "empower" clients by having them and their families take on more tasks, such as cooking and bathing, and more responsibility for "basic physiotherapy and other simple medical procedures." It intends to network with other CCACs "in order to determine which practices are the most effective and cost-efficient." According to Mary Anne Baker, the CCAC's executive director, "The new buzzword around here is 'added value.' What is the 'added value' of this or that to the people we service? That is the question we now ask. It's actually quite good. It gives you direction and helps you focus on your priorities."[37]

"Added value" of course can be used metaphorically or in the way economists use it. It is not clear from the quotation which meaning Ms. Baker intended. But there seems to be a trend towards pressuring nurses to "improve productivity." The Registered Nurses' Association of Ontario reports that CCAC case managers have been adopting very restrictive approaches "in the development and approval of care plans." It claims that "case managers require care plans that focus on nursing tasks and do not address the holistic needs, such as education and psycho-social needs of clients and their families; approach care plan development solely from a cost-control perspective; strictly interpret eligibility criteria in developing the care plan; restrict nurses to issues directly related to initial diagnosis."[38] The eclipsing of the holistic, bio-social approach in favour of a heightened division of labour based on a fragmenting medical approach is characteristic of several branches of medicine. Its impact has been documented in the restructuring of hospitals.[39] The restrictive interpretation of eligibility criteria is illustrated by a recent incident in Windsor.

In February 2000, the Windsor-Essex CCAC was in the news after a blind 81-year-old widower, whose homemaking service had been cut off, set fire to his apartment while attempting to heat some soup for himself. For five years, John Paun had been receiving a daily one-hour visit from a homemaker, who cleaned his home and cooked his dinner. The CCAC had decided that Mr. Paun was no longer eligible for this service, however, because he was still able to dress and bathe himself. After four days on his own, Mr. Paun had decided to try to cook for himself. "What am I supposed to do, starve? I have to eat," he said, after the firefighters had come to put out the fire.[40] After the incident, the CCAC restored some service to Mr. Paun. Legal Assistance of Windsor also appealed the CCAC's decision to cease providing him with service.[41]

The case is interesting, not just because it illustrates the limitations of the eligibility criteria for care, but also because it calls attention to the downloading of costs involved. On the one hand, paid work is replaced by unpaid work. After Mr. Paun's story became public, dozens of people telephoned to offer help on a voluntary basis. A local Anglican church also set out to recruit volunteers to provide the services which had been cut.[42] Secondly, costs are downloaded from the province to the municipality. In the wake of the Paun case, it came to light that Windsor's social services department "has been called upon to provide homemaking services when clients are cut off by the CCAC, which has resulted in a waiting list of 192 people. (...) But the city's home support program, which has an annual budget of $60,000, was only meant to provide top-up services for people in need who have reached the maximum number of hours available to them through the CCAC."⁴³

Once again, the cascading nature of privatization is in evidence here:
- the Ministry of Health sets out to be more businesslike and "downsize its operation"; in the name of using resources most appropriately, it puts pressure on institutions to offer the cheapest form of care, notably by shifting patients from acute care to chronic care, from the latter to long-term care facilities, and from all three to the home;
- the Ministry of Health slashes funding to hospitals, forcing them to ration their resources, change their management and re-examine their care practices;
- meanwhile, hospitals are already involved in an ongoing process of re-engineering of their own and are using technological innovation to treat more and more patients on an out-patient basis, as well as sending patients home sooner;
- more and more people need to rely on home care, but home care too is rationed and governed by the logic of "using resources where they are needed most": individuals have to rely more and more on municipal government, voluntary organizations, neighbours and kin—and ultimately just on themselves.

Needs are not being met, especially among the neediest citizens

The upshot, therefore, is further privatization: those with money may purchase additional services privately; others may simply do without. Everyone must rely more on informal care, if they are fortunate enough to have friends, neighbours or family to provide it. According to data published in the *Canada Health Monitor* in 1998:

> at least half of the users of community services, or their care givers, are paying themselves for all or part of their community services, either directly or through insurance. Of this 50 percent of the users of community services who are paying themselves: 16 percent pay up to $20 a week, 28 percent pay between $20 and $40 a week, 40 percent pay between $40 and $70 a week, and 18 percent pay more than $70 a week. (...) About 20 percent of care givers reported that the person for whom they were caring did without some services, because they could not afford them.⁴⁴

Moreover, Statistics Canada reports that "formal support has been widely used to *complement* rather than substitute for informal sources." Most needs are met through informal care. *But there are very significant inequalities in terms of income and gender*:

The prevalence of need and unmet need for personal assistance was greater among lower-income and less educated seniors, compared with those who lived in higher-income households and had more education. As well, seniors with lower incomes were more dependent on formal services than were higher-incomes seniors. Thus, without formal support, socio-economic disparities in unmet needs might have been wider, with a consequent worsening of health for those not receiving necessary care.[45]

And yet, that relative absence of formal support is precisely the situation today. *Unmet need is also gender-specific.* While among men, "the prevalence of unmet need varied little by socio-economic status and was lower than that for women in each category," among women lower levels of income and education were correlated with greater degrees of unmet need.[46] It is probable that men's needs are more likely to be met because they are looked after by women, but that the latter cannot as readily count on someone to look after them.

Re-engineering home care:
The introduction of managed competition

The Conservative government introduced a mechanism for selecting home care providers and allocating public funds in the sector that was a radical departure for Ontario. Very much in keeping with the alternative service delivery model, it has:

- severed the policy and financial functions from the allocation and contracting functions: the province sets home care policy and the overall budget envelopes, but has vested the power of allocating public monies and selecting provider agencies in formally autonomous corporations, the Community Care Access Centres (CCACs);
- severed the general functions of purchasing services, co-ordination, assessment and case management, from the specific functions of service delivery (shift nursing, home support, occupational therapy, etc.): the CCAC does the former, and is required to contract out the latter to non-profit and for-profit agencies;
- established a model whereby the CCAC acts as a broker and follows a formal procedure for tendering services, receiving and sorting bids, selecting winners and managing competition;
- has thrown the competition open to all: non-profits, for-profits, established agencies and brand new ones.

This process of privatizing much of home care, though recent, has already had a visible impact on the sector.

In this section, we shall look at the origin of the brokerage model, at the brokers and providers, and at the competitive bidding process, before discussing some of the key issues raised by managed competition: (1) assessing and ensuring the quality and continuity of care, and (2) the drawbacks of for-profit service provision in community care.

Origin of the brokerage model

Home care services developed unevenly and along a number of different paths in Ontario after the Second World War. The 1958 *Homemakers and Nurses Services Act* "established programs for homemaking and home-nursing care to be cost-shared 50/50 by the province and municipalities, and to be operated under the discretion of the municipalities." A decade later, senior governments' share went up to 80 percent and coverage was extended to other services, such as respite care.[47] Municipalities provided home care services directly, and also availed themselves of the services of non-profit agencies such as the Victorian Order of Nurses and the Red Cross. In the 1960s, the Ministry of Health added its own range of home-care services, first for convalescing acute-care patients, then later also for chronic-care patients. The Ministry of Community and Social Services also began providing or supporting services such as meals-on-wheels and home support.[48]

While there were many services, they were not equally or evenly available or accessible. There was a perceived lack of co-ordination and integration, not just among community services, but also between the latter and other parts of the health care system, such as hospitals. Standards and costs were seen as varying widely from one part of the province to another. There were reportedly inequities in the way home care programs were funded. The agencies that provided home care were "expected to raise 30 percent of their approved budgets from client charges, donations and fund-raising."[49] Yet, there were considerable differences between both the agencies and the different regions of the province, as a result of which some could raise much more money than others. A policy paper published by David Peterson's Liberal government in 1989 stated:

> [N]o single agency has either the mandate or the resources to conduct comprehensive functional assessments or to fully co-ordinate the delivery of a wide range of services for the elderly. Similarly, no agency has sole responsibility for monitoring changes in the individual's situation and arranging modifications in the range, type or intensity of services provided as the person's needs

change. Consequently, some senior citizens never have the benefit of a comprehensive assessment and others, or their families, go from agency to agency in an effort to obtain appropriate services. There is a need not only to improve access but also to provide a more comprehensive approach to the delivery of community health and social services.[50]

The Peterson government proposed the institution of "one-stop shopping," in the form of "Service Access Organizations," agencies that would broker services by non-governmental providers, while providing referrals, information, assessment and co-ordination. The role of volunteers in the system was greatly stressed.[51] In November 1991, Bob Rae's NDP government published a discussion document entitled *Redirection of Long-Term Care and Support Services in Ontario*. The document took up the idea of creating "service co-ordinator agencies" (SCA), which would act "as vehicles for assessing, brokering, and making referrals to other types of services." They would not provide services themselves, but be "brokers, purchasing services from other agencies in their communities on the basis of their assessment of a client's needs." However, in ongoing consultations with the public, the government concluded that the brokerage model was not the correct approach, because it would create a new layer of bureaucracy, hinder the improvement of the quality of service delivery, and fail to address the crucial issue of integrating health and social services. The latter was considered particularly important, both so that individuals could obtain appropriate care and services, and to avoid financial discrimination between health and community support services. The Ontario Community Support Association and the Senior Citizens' Consumer Alliance, for example, rejected the brokerage model, arguing "that service be delivered through 'comprehensive multi-service organizations,' which would be planned by integrated health and social services long-term-care committees of District Health Councils."[52]

In 1994, the Rae government passed Bill 173, "An Act Respecting Long-Term Care." The objective of Bill 173 was to streamline and enhance home care and long-term care in Ontario by establishing some 200 Multi-Service Agencies (MSA). The latter would have provided a single access point to all home and health services for independent living.

The MSAs were to deliver most home care services themselves directly. Any purchase of services from an outside agency, whether for-profit or non-profit, was to be "the exception, not the standard." A ceiling of ten percent of the MSAs' budgets was established for the purchase of any services from commercial agencies. Furthermore, those agencies purchasing less than 10 percent of their budgets' worth of services from commercial firms, would see their contracting to external agencies frozen at their existing levels. All services would be provided on a strictly non-profit basis, with existing non-profit agencies being absorbed into Integrated Homemaker Program sites.[53]

While Bill 173 was welcomed by many groups, such as the Ontario Coalition of Senior Citizens and the Senior Citizens' Alliance for Long-Term Care, some non-profit service providers (such as the Victorian Order of Nurses, the St. Elizabeth Visiting Nurses' Association, and the Red Cross) had opposed it, on the grounds that it would jeopardize their very existence, by consolidating services offered by some 1,200 different agencies and their branches under the umbrella of the new MSAs. One of the Harris government's first actions on coming to power in 1995 was to shelve the plan to establish the MSAs.

In January 1996, Conservative Health Minister Jim Wilson announced his intention to rationalize what he called the "dog's breakfast" of long-term care by establishing forty-three *Community Care Access Centres* (CCACs), with initial budgets amounting to $1.1 billion.[54] The CCACs were meant to offer the single access point to services proposed by the Liberals and promised by the NDP government's Bill 173. However, the NDP plan had called for Multi-Service Agencies to deliver a large proportion of services themselves. The Conservatives by contrast opted for the brokerage model already considered and rejected by the NDP. The CCACs were to play a role as brokers, funders and co-ordinators, but not to deliver services themselves. Instead, they were to manage competition between a variety of outside agencies. The rationale was that the separation of purchaser and supplier in a managed competition setting would lead to closer measurement of costs and benefits and therefore greater efficiency.[55] Services could continue being offered by traditional non-profit providers, such as the VON, but for-profit and non-profit corporations would now be allowed to bid on contracts. Some of the latter were local companies set up by nurses and other practitioners previously employed in the public sector. Others were larger Canadian or foreign corporations (e.g. Comcare Health Services, Para-Med Health Services, or Olsten Health Services). Some of the CCACs were completely new organizations, while others were built upon existing home-care programs. The latter were given a deadline (late 1999/early 2000) to divest themselves of any direct service provision.

A profile of the brokers

The CCACs are incorporated as non-profit organizations; 59 percent of them are registered charities, while 7 percent are public charitable foundations.[56] However, CCACs are entirely financed by the provincial government. Although about half report receiving some membership dues and/or donations from individuals, these represented in all cases a negligible proportion of their revenues. Only one CCAC reported doing any fund-raising.[57]

Tightly bound to the Ministry of Health and Long-Term Care by detailed contracts, the CCACs are very much creatures of the provincial government. They are confined by rigid budgets allocated by the province, from which they receive all their money. The creation of these organizations has resulted in the *privatization* of important information about home care. Even though the CCACs are entirely financed by the provincial government, the latter will not divulge key information about their activities, deeming it to be private and confidential. A letter from the Ministry of Health and Long-Term Care responding to a request for information from the Canadian Centre for Policy Alternatives states:

> I am unable to provide you with the detailed statistics on expenditures by each CCAC, due to limitations under the Freedom of Information and Protection of Privacy Act. Each CCAC is an autonomous non-profit incorporated organization which operates under a service agreement with the ministry to provide a range of services to the residents of Ontario. The detailed proprietary financial reports submitted by each CCAC to the Ministry of Health are considered to be third party financial information supplied in confidence, and as such, are not available for public release.[58]

The amounts paid to other outside agencies directly by the Ministry of Health and Long-Term Care are published every year in the *Public Accounts of Ontario*. Yet, when the payments are made through the Community Care Access Centres, they are deemed private.

Democratic governance of home care is obstructed by this lack of transparency. Because the commercial interests of competing firms are involved, the provincial government is not prepared to divulge all information about service contracts, nor are a number of CCACs (although many have revealed themselves to be very generous and helpful in giving of their time and knowledge). It is very difficult for the public to get an overall picture of who is getting the money, and how and why spending decisions are made.

It is ironic that the same provincial government which has legislated the mandatory publication of the salaries of senior civil servants, executives of crown corporations and academics, at the same time insists on the confidentiality of contracts going to non-profit and for-profit corporations in the health and home care sector. CCACs are entirely financed by the government; indeed their only role is to act as agents of the government in disbursing monies for home care. How public money is spent should be transparent. One of the effects of the creation of these "autonomous non-profit incorporated organizations" is the privatization of information on how tax money is being spent. Ironically, while the province cites the need to protect the interests of the provider agencies, some of them have expressed frustration at the secrecy of the tendering process.[59]

A profile of the provider agencies

As noted above, there are dozens of non-profit and for-profit agencies across Ontario that provide home-care services. In the Ottawa-Carleton area, for example, a walk through the yellow pages turns up over a dozen names under the rubric "home health services" and some twenty names under "nurses." These include some Ottawa-based agencies, as well as the local branches of corporations that operate across Ontario, or even across Canada and North America: Bayshore HealthCare, Saint Elizabeth Health Care, VHA Health and Home Support, Para-Med Home Health Care, We Care Home Health Services, and the Victorian Order of Nurses. Of course, not all of these agencies are receiving public funds under contract with the CCAC.

A recent study published by the federal government states that "there are at least 663 agencies providing home care services in Canada, with 93 percent of agencies receiving some government funding and just over 50 percent receiving all of their funding from government sources."[60] Of these agencies, 67.1 percent are independent; the rest are branches or franchises of provincial, national or international for-profit and non-profit organizations such as the Victorian Order of Nurses, Saint-Elizabeth Health Care, We Care, Comcare, Para-Med, Olsten, and the Red Cross. Some three-quarters of the agencies offer a range of services that extends beyond home care. The median number of staff is 42; the median number of clients served is 1,475.

The independent agencies are small and locally based. These could include small businesses which have carved out a niche for themselves by selling services to private customers. An example is Retire-at-Home Services Inc., a company founded by a nurse, Irene Martin, with offices in Ottawa and Nepean, Ontario. For such a firm, preserving a reputation for outstanding service is crucial to building its share of the private market.

Small agencies can be found in the market for publicly-funded contracts, too, although it would appear that they tend to be concentrated *geographically* in urban centres—especially Toronto, but also some regional centres—and *sectorally* (e.g., home support services for ethnic minorities; also, some agencies formed by therapists divested by CCACs).

In nursing and homemaking, which absorb the lion's share of home care budgets, the field of publicly funded services is completely dominated by a half-dozen agencies. In nursing, these are the Victorian Order of Nurses (VON), Para-Med Health Services, Comcare, Saint-Elizabeth Health Care, and Gentiva Health Services (formerly Olsten). In homemaking, they are the Red Cross, Para-Med, Comcare, Gentiva, Bayshore, Saint-Elizabeth Health Care.

VON, Saint-Elizabeth Health Care and the Red Cross are charitable organizations with a history of community service that spans the 20th century. The others are private for-profit companies. Para-Med is a wholly-owned subsidiary of Extendicare, a company based in Markham, Ontario, which ranks among the largest North American operators of long-term care and assisted-living facilities for the elderly. Its shares are traded on the stock exchanges in Toronto, Montreal and New York. It runs 323 facilities, with over 30,000 beds, in Canada, the United States and Great Britain. Para-Med has 47 branch offices in Ontario, Alberta and British Columbia. Comcare was founded a quarter of a century ago by the Nickerson family of St. Catharines, Ontario. It is active in Ontario, Quebec, New Brunswick, Nova Scotia, Alberta and British Columbia. It is based in London, Ontario. Comcare was acquired in 1997 by Medcare, a subsidiary of Gamma-Dynacare, one of the three multinational corporations that dominate the laboratory testing market in Ontario (see Chapter 2). Gentiva was until March 2000 a subsidiary of Long-Island-based Olsten Corporation, a giant firm that operates 1500 offices in 14 countries on three continents.[61] As an independent corporation, Gentiva remains huge, with $1.5 billion in revenues in 1999 and a major stake in sectors such as pharmaceuticals and home care.[62]

The managed competition process

Competitive bidding in home care in Ontario is an extremely formal, rigid process which unfolds over the better part of a year. The CCAC begins by soliciting expressions of interest and statements of qualifications from potential bidders. Once it has studied the submissions it receives in reply, it invites the agencies which exhibit a given level of qualifications to respond to a request for proposals (RFP). Some of these requests-for-proposals are posted on the internet or in newspapers. Most are posted on Merx, the central point through which public-sector agencies tender service contracts.

In some cases, the committee which assesses the proposals first looks at them strictly from the point of view of the quality of service they promise, without any knowledge of the prices the agencies quote. Only once a short-list of the highest-quality bids has been established does the committee take cognizance of the prices and choose the winning bidders. However, it was not possible to determine whether this was the practice everywhere. The Ontario Home Health Care Providers' Association recommends this as a "best practice" in its March 1999 position paper on the CCACs' competitive bidding process.[63] This suggests that it was *not* a universal practice at least until then.

Bidders are supplied with a sometimes book-length manual detailing the exact form a bid must take, the type of contents it is expected to include, and the dates and stages of the process. No delays are allowed. Missing a deadline by even minutes or hours means exclusion from the competition. Proposals from provider agencies must be comprehensive documents that provide assurances that they have the logistical, administrative and technological ability not only to deliver the full range of required services, but also that they can interact with the CCAC in prescribed ways in matters such as billing (not only must the latter for example be timely, etc., but the agency must guarantee that it has the computer hardware and software needed "to interface with the CCAC's information system for purposes of direct billing"). Bidders have also been asked to supply the CCAC with detailed information about the remuneration, training and qualifications of their care-giving staff, about standards of practice, codes of ethics, procedures for responding to clients' complaints, about ways of assessing and coming to grips with the cultural and linguistic needs of service users, etc.

Although the Ministry of Health and Long-Term Care provided CCACs with a template to guide them in designing their RFPs, they do not appear to have developed any uniform or consistent model. This has given rise to much criticism, from both non-profit and for-profit agencies and their associations. As the Registered Nurses' Association complained:

> Most CCACs did not indicate in RFPs the number of providers to be awarded volumes [of service]. Further, there was little, if any,

explanation in RFPs as to how service volumes would be allocated among successful bidders. In some instances, the entire volume was awarded to one agency. Sometimes volumes were equally divided among 2 or 3 organizations despite significant differences in price. In other situations, different volumes were awarded to multiple providers with different prices. This resulted in questions about the price/quality trade-off and the consistency of quality standards among various providers.[64]

The RFP process is also extremely arduous for the bidders. According to one informant, submitting proposals can cost an agency $10,000 to $20,000 per year. In one case, one employee worked full-time for four months writing the proposals.[65] Organizations that operate on a province-wide basis appear to have had an edge here over those in which each branch acted autonomously and depended on its own resources. The huge effort entailed by the competitive bidding process favours larger, but also more centralized, agencies which have rationalized the use of their administrative resources across Ontario.

The traditional non-profit and public service providers were sheltered from full-blown competition at first. Suppliers were guaranteed a gradually declining percentage of the volume of work they had received in 1995—90 percent in 1996, 80 percent in 1997, 70 percent in 1998. A growing share of the work was open to competition. As of April 1999, the bidding was to be thrown wide open to all potential providers. However, the implementation of this schedule has been uneven, and the RFP process had not yet been fully implemented across the province in the spring of 2000. The Hamilton-Wentworth CCAC's web site provides an example of an intended RFP schedule (see Table 4).

However, the province also built into the process a mechanism that ensured that agencies would lose some of the business in areas where they had been the sole provider. In a May 1996 document attached to the letter explaining the transition to managed competition, the Ministry of Health laid down one of the cornerstones of the new process: "A mix of service providers will be maintained in each community, wherever feasible."[66] Thus, even though agencies were protected from full competition for three years, the system was designed in such a way that no agency could any longer be the sole provider, even if it unequivocally offered the best service. The qualification "wherever feasible" was evidently meant to be an escape clause in more sparsely populated areas where the volume of service was too low to attract for-profit bidders.[67]

Table 16 illustrates the staggered implementation process and the move towards standard contract lengths, starting dates and completion times. Although the typical contract length in this example is four years, this is not the norm for all CCAC contracts. Many offer two- or three-year contracts. For example, the Wellington-Dufferin, Sarnia-Lambton, and Muskoka-Parry Sound CCACs' current contracts are for a three-year period starting in 1999.[69]

Formalizing the bidding process was supposed to define standards of quality, giving CCACs clear objectives and outcomes for which to aim. Provider agencies were obliged to explain how they ensured the quality of their service, and CCACs had to determine how to evaluate

Table 16
Hamilton-Wentworth CCAC—intended RFP schedule (March 2000)

Service	Percentage	Contract start	Contract end		Contract length
Homemaking	30	Nov. 1998	March 2000		1 year, 5 months
	100	April 2000	March 2004		4 years
	100	April 2004	March 2008		4 years
Nursing	30	Nov. 1998	March 2001	*	2 years, 5 months
	20	July 1999	March 2003	*	3 years, 9 months
	50	July 1999	March 2002		2 years, 9 months
	30	April 2001	March 2003		2 years
	50	April 2002	March 2006		4 years
	50	April 2003	March 2007		4 years
Therapy	25	October 1999	March 2004	**	4 years, 6 months
	75	October 2000	March 2004		4 years
	100	April 2004	March 2008		4 years
Medical supplies	100	April 1998	March 2001	***	3 years
	100	April 2001	April 2005		4 years
IV	100	April 1998	March 2001	***	3 years
	100	April 2001	April 2005		4 years
Medical equipment	100	April 1998	March 2001	***	3 years
	100	April 2001	April 2005		4 years

* 12-month extension; ** 18-month extension; *** 24-month extension.

Notes
1. RFP process will typically begin in September for April contract start.
2. Nursing contract extensions:
   - St. Elizabeth Nursing has accepted a 12-month extension
   - Olsten has accepted a 12-month extension
   - To be determined: 20% from amongst the E/W/M contracts
3. Medical Supplies and IV extension:
   - Caremark has accepted a 12-month extension; has been offered and accepted another 12-month extension
4. Medical Equipment extension:
   - Shoppers has accepted a 12-month extension; has been offered and accepted another 12-month extension
5. Therapy extension:
   - Recently awarded contracts may be extended a further 18 months

Source: Hamilton-Wentworth CCAC[68]

the proposals and to score bids in a fair way. The access centres also had to establish a way of weighting quality and price.

To be sure, the Ontario Ministry of Long-Term Care created a template, based on a mix of quality and cost, for determining who should receive contracts to deliver home care services. Each CCAC could then adapt this template to its own situation and needs. In York Region, for example, the assessment process attributed slightly greater weight to service quality (60 per cent) than to cost (40 per cent). The CCAC in the Waterloo region reportedly had a 70:30 quality/price ratio to begin with, but changed it to 90:10, downplaying cost and emphasizing quality[70] (see Table 17). However, given limited, inelastic budgets, and rapidly

Table 17	
The balance between quality and cost in CCACs' RFP processes	
CCAC	Quality/cost
1	80/20
2	75/25
3	80/20
4	90/10 (direct services), 75/25 (therapies), 25/75 (supplies, equipment)
5	70/25/5 (5% = benefits provided to employees by service providers)
6	75/25
7	80/20
8	75-25 or 85/15 (according to RFP)
9	75/25
10	80/20
11	85/15
12	Must hit minimum threshold before cost is considered
13	90/10
14	85/15
14	80/20
15	80/20
16	80/20
17	95/20 (95=80+ 5 for site visit + 10 for case study)
18	90/10
19	75/25
20	100/0
21	70/30
22	75/25 (nursing, personal support) 60/40 equipment
23	90/10
24	81.7/18.3
25	80/20
26	80/20
27	80/20
28	75/25
29	90/10, 80/20

Source: *CCPA Fall Survey of CCACs*

growing demand, there was clearly considerable pressure on CCACs to contain costs.

"Measuring" quality

The great conundrum for all institutions implementing a competitive process is (1) how to design contracts so that they will yield services of high quality; and (2) how to assess the impact of treatment or care on patients. One of the driving forces in management theories and practices since the industrial revolution has been the attempt to define and design all the tasks to be accomplished by or for a business in a *quantifiable* way, on the motto that *if you can measure it, you can control it*. Yet, though *quality* is one of the great buzzwords in business—one need only think of how every organization, not least in health care, has embraced "total quality management" and "continuous quality improvement"—it is hard to get around the fact that "measuring quality" is an oxymoron. By definition, quality is that which is not measurable. The way around this is to find proxies—measurable phenomena that are held to indicate whether quality is present or not.

This is the paradox of modern management generally: managers need to control their employees or sub-contractors, and can only do so by making them perform standardized tasks with "measurable outcomes." Contracting works best when the goods or services to be delivered can be defined and measured with great precision. Examples of such goods could include materials used in industry, such as lengths of steel cable, tubing or bricks. In home care, they could include the supply of bandages, accessories for incontinence care, or toilet commodes. A strict commercial contracting regime works much less efficiently when the goods and services to be delivered are not easily defined, quantified and measured, or when the outcomes are uncertain.

Research services are a case where outcomes cannot be predicted with absolute certainty. One may contract with a researcher to find original data about a given social phenomenon. This might prove a straightforward task. But the research process may establish that there is no or little previous research on the subject, and that the sources of empirical evidence are absent, closed, or unreliable. In such cases, the research may well prove fruitless. Failure to provide the requested data in such instances does not demonstrate failure to live up to the contract.

When contracting for *research*, it is not possible to require the researcher(s) to reach a predetermined conclusion. By definition, research is an open, truth-seeking activity. To impose a given conclusion on it ahead of time is to pervert it and transform it into a propaganda exercise. No genuine research contract therefore could be required to arrive at a predetermined conclusion. Its outcome is inherently uncertain. Failure to confirm the initial hypothesis could never be construed as failure to live up to the terms of the contract.

Similarly, outcomes in health care, indeed human services generally, cannot easily be predicted or guaranteed. Trying to ensure the highest quality of care is a matter of some methodological complexity. In home care, the assessment of the care needed can involve the work of several professionals (physician, case manager, visiting nurse, therapist) working within the frameworks established by their respective scientific disciplines, by their clinical and administrative practices (governed by professional colleges), and by the institutions to which they are attached (e.g., CCAC, provider agency, hospital, etc.). In addition, monitoring the actual care provided in the home presents enormous difficulties. For these reasons, "there are very important information imperfections in markets for services with outcomes which are uncertain, technically complex, infrequently produced, of long gestation and embodied in the characteristics of the users themselves."[71]

There are two ways of addressing these issues. One is to "attempt to specify in great detail, in advance, all the measurable dimensions of quality (but this increases the administrative burden of specification and monitoring)." The other strategy is to "rely upon known and trusted suppliers and/or agree upon common standards (but this may result in a lack of competition)." Often, "purchasers and providers make contracts which stress inputs or processes rather than outputs or outcomes."[72] Such was the traditional approach in the public service. In recent years, partly in connection with the "reinventing government" trend, there has been a movement to emphasize "outcomes." This has spawned a considerable amount of effort to define and develop new indicators. The academic study of evaluation has also grown considerably.

Everything hinges, then, on how quality is defined. Does it mean the efficiency with which services are performed? Or does it include other considerations apart from the actual service, such as the identity of the service provider? As the Registered Nurses' Association of Ontario put it: "The RFP relies on proxy measures of quality, such as number of RNs and RPNs, supervision ratios, continuing education programs, quality improvement and risk management programs."[73]

While confident in her agency's ability to compete and believing that all bidders in her area are treated impartially, the executive director of a non-profit agency expressed concern to me that the RFP process takes place essentially on paper. Winning the contract seems to consist very much in having the skills to write good proposals. What this means is that firms that offer inferior services, but are better at self-presentation, may be getting the contracts. The non-profits have had to work on developing the skills in self-advertisement that go with a competitive market environment. This is obviously true within the bidding process itself, where having a long history of service within the community no longer necessarily weighs much in the balance. Given the superior resources some large, for-profit firms have, their greater ability to put together proposals that are good on paper may outweigh the greater excellence of non-profits as actual service providers. There is awareness of this among CCACs. As one CCAC CEO explained:

> Quality is very hard to evaluate in the RFP process. We struggled from the beginning with how to evaluate quality in actual fact, not just on the basis of what is on paper—somebody could be very good at writing proposals, but not be very good on the front line of providing services. We did build in some simple mechanisms. One was a site visit, but only to the offices to get a feeling for the people and the organization and to look first-hand at their quality-monitoring mechanism, how they record complaints and what they do with them. A next step might be to make some home visits, with some clients. The other thing we've done is a case study: all the providers are given the story in advance and are asked to come and make a presentation before a panel of three to explain how they would handle that case. They have the case in advance, they have had time to prepare, and they know they will be heard by three judges. It was very interesting: the range of responses was enormous. There were some companies that sent a person who had only been employed by them for two weeks; of course, she couldn't do a very good job of presenting the case. Another firm sent fourteen of their top people from across the nation. Others were in between. During the process, we stopped them in their tracks and changed an element of the story, so that we could see how they think on their feet. In real life, that's what they would be faced with. We tried hard to build in a few things that would help us assess more than the paper exercise.[74]

Considerable ingenuity may go into structuring an interview process in such as way as to yield some picture of how an agency would *potentially* react to various situations. But this is still a long way from monitoring actual practice.

The Ontario Home Health Care Providers' Association in its brief in fact called for a consistent *auditing* process to ensure the "provision of the promised quality of service at the promised time, within the submitted price."[75] But desirable as such an audit would be, it is still based on the assumption that the competitive process and contract can define and ensure the services needed and the desired quality of service. To be sure, they can specify that an agency will provide x number of professional home visits or homemaking hours, perform y number of tasks while there, do so on agreed-upon dates and at the quoted price. But that is the mere shell of home care, not its true substance. As a provider agency executive put it: "Managed competition provides rigour to piecemealing out the work, understanding in very simplistic way what you are in fact bidding for."[76] It is about mere *quantity*, not *quality*. The latter is much more a matter of *trust*—in agencies' commitments, in their reputation, in the professionalism of their staff.

Several executives of CCACs and provider agencies I spoke with saw the existence of explicit *standards* as an important difference between the new regime of competitive bidding and the situation that existed before. The implication seemed to be that the brokers and providers had been obliged to conceptualize and make explicit aspects of their practice which had perhaps been taken for granted or dealt with on an ad hoc basis before. Yet, no one seems to be saying that visiting nurses are more professional now than they were previously. It would seem that the standards are more administrative than they are clinical.

But even on the administrative level, the way the system is set up raises doubts. For example, Saint-Elizabeth Health Care, a leading non-profit home care provider, has developed an interesting new information technology tool, *e-care*, with assistance from Health Canada. Thanks to this software package, diabetic patients can be advised and educated about their condition, while communicating regularly, even daily, with their nurse, and being monitored by her/him. Patient and nurse have more sustained and useful contact, yet fewer home visits are needed.[77] Yet, the payment system is set up in such a way that the provider agencies are paid by the visit. It is not hard to see that, in cutting down on the number of visits, *e-care* eats into Saint-Elizabeth's billing potential. There is a clear disincentive to develop this kind of new approach. Such innovation is what non-profit associations are meant to do; but the system's built-in incentives militate against it.

Managed competition and the undermining of trust between agencies

By their very nature, community health services, then, "are extremely difficult to specify, 'contractualize' and monitor, and are also highly dependent on inter-professional and inter-agency collaboration. They thus require substantial amounts of trust in the professional discretion of providers." The purchasers, providers and users of home care services must develop a "high-trust relationship," in which participants:

- "share (or have similar) ends and values;
- "have a diffuse sense of long-term obligation;
- "offer support without calculating the cost or expecting an immediate return;
- "communicate freely and openly with one another;
- "are prepared to trust the other and risk their own fortunes in the other party; and
- "give the benefit of the doubt in relation to motives and goodwill if there are problems."[78]

Trust is crucial in home care. It develops in networks of agencies, professionals and service users.

Unfortunately, research suggests that market relationships transform those networks, eroding trust and collaboration, and replacing them with guardedness and competition.[79] In the resulting "low-trust relationships," participants:

- "have divergent goals and interests;
- "have explicit expectations which must be reciprocated through balanced exchanges;
- "carefully calculate the costs and benefits of any concession made;
- "restrict and screen communications in their own separate interests;
- "attempt to minimize their dependence on the other's discretion; and
- "are suspicious about mistakes or failures, attributing them to ill-will or default and invoke sanctions."[80]

The nature of home care work is such that outcomes are difficult to define and formalize. Performance and quality are difficult to measure. Trust is essential. Yet the contracting process puts aside this element of trust in favour of a very different notion of quality, rooted in imperatives of financial accountability and control. Furthermore, the market mechanism, with its regular RFPs, is driven by, and drives, short-term planning about immediate outcomes and cost-containment. Yet, improving health requires long-range planning, and continuity of practice and care.[81]

A CCAC executive I interviewed expressed discomfort with this feature of the competitive process. On the one hand, from the point of view of *producing* the services, the overriding objective must be the greatest good of the people who use the servive. This should mean that the various providers should work in teams and share information about their work methods and their best practices. Yet the competitive environment by its very nature makes organizations reluctant to share information about their initiatives and best practices with each other:

> Competition means that the continuity cannot be guaranteed. The process can be made predictable, but not the result. There will be winners and losers. That doesn't respect the client's need for continuity. We've set up a system that goes against that value right from the outset. It is a tricky issue for me, this RFPing. I look ahead to when we have to do this again: we'll have invested three years in getting to know the agencies, in building relationships, in working really hard on quality issues and improving the service, and we'll have to go into another RFP with no guarantee of the results. We'll have to live with the latter, even if we don't like them, as long as we've been true to our process. What if it changes? What if we have some new providers in the mix? We'll be back at square one, having to build relationships, learn to work together, etc. As a human-service business, I am not sure that the benefits in quality and cost will outweigh the difficulties in relationship-building, trust and communication.[82]

Similarly, an executive of a provider agency I spoke with described the relationship between the provider agencies and the home care program before managed competition as one of *friendly competition*. Because the provider agencies did not fear the loss of contract and therefore potentially their own demise, they planned and operated much more in partnership, consulting much more, and sharing information and resources, notably with respect to education, program-development expertise, and so on. As non-profit organizations, their goal was to maximize the benefit to the public through sharing, as opposed to trying to be more productive.[83]

The home care system that existed before managed competition seems to correspond to the notion of "relational contracts," in which "services are jointly developed, there are highly specific assets, undertakings cannot be fully specified in advance, and mechanisms are sought to preserve long-term relationships."[84] Instead of the secret, opaque, competitive RFP quasi-market, there appears to have been a *network* of providers. Networks are associated with such values as altruism, loyalty, solidarity, reciprocity, trust[85]—values which the non-profit sector is widely held to be likely to encourage. As Flynn, Williams and Pickard put it: "A network structure is often preferred to secure mutual reliance and support, especially where there is a need for trust in the reliability and quality of the product or service supplied. Networks, Powell argued, are valuable for the exchange of commodities whose value cannot be precisely determined, such as 'know-how' and other services which are not easily priced or traded through the market."[86]

Managed competition undermines continuity of service—loss of continuity undermines the trust between provider and user

From the point of view of those *using* the services, the most important thing is *continuity of service*. Because of the very personal and intimate nature of the work of nurses, personal- support workers and therapists, it is very, very important for providers and users to build relationships of trust with each other. This is possible only if the same providers see the same clients on a long-term, regular basis. This issue is crucial in the eyes of home care experts, including several CCAC managers I spoke with, who exhibited considerable ambivalence about the new regime, lamenting the loss of continuity for the service users. But when asked what the solution was, several of my informants threw the question back at me: what is the alternative? The multi-service agency? Nobody wanted that, they said. So now we have managed competition. (Of course, many people did want the multi-service agencies.) Yet, as one CCAC executive said to me:

> When a parent stands up and says to the CCAC: "I've been a client of yours for six years and I've been telling you what's important to me, and how you're operating now tells me you're disregarding everything I told you," it doesn't feel very good. It's not good enough for the CCAC to say that it's been going by the rules, so everything is OK. There's something wrong. People are not just standing up for VON or other agencies that have lost contracts. They are giving voice to the fact that they are the clients and that the most important thing to them is continuity of the worker. How do we include the will of our clients in our processes? That's what's missing in our process, and I presume in everybody's. Clients were not asked at any point in our process to evaluate the companies. It's tricky, because vulnerable people may be reluctant to speak out for fear of jeopardizing their care. From an ethical perspective, we have to get some sort of popular input into the monitoring of the quality.[87]

This once again raises the issue of democracy. In the competitive model, the "macro" decisions about care all get taken between the managers at the CCAC and the managers in the provider agencies. The actual workers and the recipients of care only come into the picture later, when the "micro" decisions are made. But even there, the CCAC and provider-agency managers are still calling the shots. What is needed is a way of giving a lot more say to the front-line workers and the users of the services. In a context of care, this means breaking down the barriers that separate, divide and isolate purchasers and providers, workers and users.

Challenging the purchaser/provider split

In this respect, one CCAC executive I interviewed compared the competitive model unfavourably to the multi-service-agency model as it exists in Quebec, and might have in Ontario:

> There's some theory that supports the role of brokers, but I'm not sure... It would be interesting to compare the two models. [The MSA model here would be on the lines of Quebec, where the agency does not just do case management, but has the front-line providers as well.] In Quebec, we had very little to do with private providers, most of the providers were our own, the only ones who weren't, that we took on as contractors, were about half of the homemaking staff. That was a historical thing: half the homemakers were our own, the other half were contracted out. Over the years, we had such problems with the contractees that we had to have a full-time case manager monitoring our relationship with them, to make sure the right people were in the homes and that the appropriate services were being provided. The price we paid the agency was half what we paid our own workers, so imagine what they paid their own homemakers, less than half of what we paid ours. We found over the years that we could control the quality better by having our own homemakers. Each year we reduced the amount of our contracting out and increased the work we gave our own homemakers. They were well paid, would on their own initiative go out and improve their education, they stayed with us for a long time, they built a solid relationship with the nurses and therapists going into the home, and worked in the same building as the case manager. I am biased, having worked in that milieu and seen it work well. Our struggle is: how can we have a true client-driven system, while we're in a funding-driven, competitive model?[88]

This view is shared by Evelyn Shapiro, one of the foremost authorities on home care in Canada. She argues that the advantage of publicly-*provided*, as opposed to merely publicly-*funded*, home care, is that uniting case managers, resource co-ordinators and front-line workers in the same organization allows for much greater formal and informal communication and team work, as well as greater continuity. The people who need and use the services benefit greatly from the better co-operation and continuity of care.[89]

However, *how* the public sector provides the service may vary. The CLSC model is one option, but it is also possible to envisage networks of non-profit organizations working closely with statutory agencies. There is a considerable body of theoretical work that supports the role of non-profit organizations in the provision of health and social services.[90] At their best, non-profits are regarded as closer to the community, more cost-effective, exceptionally good at recognizing new needs, able to respond quickly and efficiently to social problems, extremely flexible and innovative, able to take risks, promote change and advocate on behalf of particular groups.[91] Governments must, however, be present "to provide universal and integrated planning, to set and monitor standards, to achieve equity and social justice through resource allocation, and to preserve democratic control."[92] In this regard, it will be interesting to follow the social economy experiment under way in Quebec, in which community organizations and co-operatives offer a range of home care services. These experiments have been highly controversial, with some observers seeing them as vehicles of privatization and others as engines of emancipation. Whichever direction they end up taking, they will likely yield valuable lessons for democratic re-organization of community care.

Why not for-profits?

The role of for-profit enterprises in human services has been the object of criticism at a number of levels. One of the major issues is what is known as *contract failure*:

> The central notion here is that for some goods and services, such as care for the aged, the purchaser is not the same as the consumer. In these circumstances, the normal mechanisms of the market—which involve consumer choice on the basis of adequate information—do not obtain. Consequently, some proxy has to be created to offer the purchaser a degree of assurance that the goods and services being purchased meet adequate standards of quality and quantity. The non-profit form, in this theory, provides that

proxy. Unlike for-profit businesses, which are motivated by profit and therefore might be tempted to betray the trust of a purchaser who is not the recipient of what he buys, non-profit firms are in business for more charitable purposes and may therefore be more worthy of trust.[93]

Advocates of the market model argue that for-profits are responsive to the consumer. But in home care, the consumer is not the purchaser; the broker is—and here the contract failure argument would apply.

Should one conclude from this that the best system is one under which individual users shop around for the best care? No: there are compelling reasons for not opting for a system where individuals must purchase their own care.

- Only a few people can afford to pay out of pocket. To avoid a multi-tier system and retain universality, everyone must have access to equally high-quality, publicly funded services.
- Users do not all have the competence to shop around, nor do they all have the necessary information about the home care market. Many users are not competent—in the worst cases, they suffer from incipient dementia or other debilitating conditions. Secondly, one cannot shop around for home care as one would for toothpaste or automobiles. Indeed, the Liberals, Conservatives and New Democrats were all agreed on the need for a single access point to long-term care. CCACs were established precisely so that users wouldn't have to find their way on their own through the labyrinth of agencies and programs on the market.
- Users are in a relation of dependency on their service providers. It is difficult for them to complain about poor service, or break off their relationship with them. Should they do so, they are left with the conundrum of finding a new agency; for many this means relying on word-of-mouth or walking through the yellow pages.
- As we saw in chapters 1 and 2, there is widespread agreement on the need to create an *integrated health care system*, in which primary, institutional and home care will not be divorced from each other, but *seamlessly* joined. Admirers of Adam Smith notwithstanding, such a system will not emerge from the myriad individual decisions of consumers trying to purchase care, any more than a national child care system has in Canada. Planning and co-ordination by governments and associated agencies are needed.
- The American experience shows that market-driven health care is more expensive. Because of the lack of central co-ordination and a single payer, huge amounts of money are squandered in adminis-

tration expenditures that could be avoided. The many payers in the United States are not able to negotiate prices as low as the provincial governments in Canada. This is one reason Americans flock to Canada in their thousands to purchase prescription drugs, which are much cheaper in Canada.

There is of course a clear alternative which avoids both the pitfalls of contract failure and the inequities and inadequacies of the *chacun pour soi* approach: public or not-for-profit provision.

The purpose of a for-profit corporation is to maximize profit. Profit maximization means that money that could be reinvested in services goes into the pockets of shareholders. Of course, the argument is that the lure of profit will lead investors to pour money into the company, enabling it to expand its operations, its sales, and therefore its services and profits. A non-profit agency, the argument goes, will not be able to achieve the same growth in sales and services.

There are two problems with this argument. First, there is no infinitely expandable market for home care services. Individuals do purchase some, but the government is the bulk purchaser. The government will not of course expand its home care infinitely in order to buy an ever-growing volume of services.

Secondly, the imperative of profit maximization ultimately overrides all other considerations, because it is the very *raison d'être* of the company.[94] The means to maximize profits include: adding on extra, lucrative services, which may be unnecessary to the patient; cream-skimming (i.e. taking on only the patients/customers whose needs are easily/ cheaply satisfied); offering less and worse service; or paying lower wages and benefits. Those who use the services will lose out.[95]

The profit motive driving private contractors is a matter of concern in home care, as it is in other human services. Writing in the *Ottawa Citizen*, April Lindgren and Michael Den Tandt quote We Care Home Health Services as saying "that franchise holders who make an initial investment of $130,000 can expect to earn pre-tax revenue of $64,000 to $149,000." They offer a telling example of the attitudes that can colour a for-profit contractor's approach:

> The potential for easy money hasn't gone unnoticed. At the We Care franchise meeting, one participant speculated about the money he could make by lining up a series of quick injections for clients. While it would take only about 15 minutes to deliver each jab, the minimum billing time for each client would be an hour at $28 to $32 per hour, he mused. At the same time, We Care general

manager Larry Gatien urged the dozen or so potential franchisees to 'be ethical'.[96]

It goes without saying that the mere injunction to behave ethically cannot carry much weight in the face of a system built on the categorical imperative to make a profit—ethical behaviour will be observed as far as it is compatible with profitability, and no further, or the business will go under. *The point is not to impugn the motives or professionalism of any specific agency or individual*[97] *, but merely to suggest that market imperatives intrinsically pit the profit motive against standards of professional care. If the latter is the paramount value—as surely no one would deny—then why set up a system that comprises competing values which threaten to undermine it continually?*

The impact of managed competition

There is a dearth of information and those who know aren't telling

We thought it would be interesting to find out whether the balance was tipping towards the private sector in terms of the share of contracts going to for-profits rather than non-profits. The first thing that needs to be said about who won and who lost in the tendering process is that this information is well hidden. The Ministry of Health and Long-Term Care will not reveal it, even though, as one CCAC CEO told me, "we're spending public money, so the public has a right to know how it's being spent."[98] The Ministry claims that this is proprietary information and as such confidential. The Ontario Association of Community Care Access Centres is presently conducting a study (to be completed in the summer of 2000) that will assess the process and impact of managed competition.

What the media has reported

In a highly-publicized case, 226 nurses and 34 clerical workers were to lose their jobs in the fall of 1999, after their employer, the Victorian Order of Nurses, lost its home-nursing contract from the Windsor-Essex CCAC to three other organizations, Saint-Elizabeth Health Care, Comcare Health Services, and American corporation Olsten Health Services. The decision was highly controversial, however, because the VON had been providing nursing services in Windsor for decades. According to the CCAC, the contracts had been awarded in a fair and rigorous manner to the agencies offering the highest-quality services.[99] However, the VON's proposal reportedly "was $7 an hour more expensive than the competing bids, largely due to higher labour costs."[100] The Canadian Union of Public Employees (CUPE), which represents the VON's Windsor-area employees, regarded the CCAC's tendering process instead as part of "the Tories' plans to privatize home care through competitive bidding, and to break union representation for community health care workers." CUPE announced that it would launch a challenge at the Ontario Labour Relations Board to claim successor rights for its threatened members. In the aftermath of the decision, most of the VON's nurses reportedly found new jobs with hospitals and nursing homes in the Windsor and Detroit areas. Meanwhile, the three agencies which had won the contract experienced shortages of nurses.[101] Rather than increase efficiency in home care, managed competition here simply seems to have helped hospitals and nursing homes out at the expense of home care.

In Simcoe County, the visiting nursing contract brought in 80 percent of the VON branch's revenue. In losing the contract in 1999, the branch was unable to continue operating. It had been providing nursing services to the area for over 75 years.[102] Overall, the VON estimated in the spring of 1999 that it had lost fourteen percent of its visiting nursing contracts that year. "We expect (...) to lose 20 to 30 percent, mostly to for-profits," Diane McLeod, the executive director of the VON's Ontario regional office was quoted as saying.[103] A former director of the VON described managed competition as "managed decline" for non-profits.[104]

On the other hand, Saint-Elizabeth Health Care, another non-profit that has existed for nearly a century, has done well. Its 1998-1999 annual report and assorted press releases indicate that it has opened new branches in Windsor, London, Waterloo, Hamilton, Clinton and Barrie as a result of winning new nursing, homemaking and therapy contracts from the CCACs in those areas.

What have we been able to find out?

1. We surveyed the Community Care Access Centres
We decided to go out and ask the CCACs themselves.
1. A December 1999-January 2000 survey asked for precise numbers of clients served, professional visits and homemaking hours provided, as well as for lists of service providers under contract in 1996-1997, 1997-1998, and 1998-1999. In addition this survey asked CCACs to indicate the percentage of the service volume provided by for-profits and non-profits respectively in each major service area.

2. An April 2000 mini-survey supplemented the lists of service providers for 1996-1999 established by the previous survey. This mini-survey also asked for a list of providers under contract from 1999 on.

The response rate for most of the questions was also good: 58.1 percent (25 CCACs). However, some of the questions were more difficult to answer. Thus, only 14 of the CCACs (32.6 percent) told us the volume of service offered respectively by for-profits and non-profits in 1998-1999, and only a half dozen or so gave us that information for 1996-1997 and 1997-1998.[105] Finally, 16 of the 43 CCACs (37.2 percent) gave us information about the agencies under contract for the period after 1999.

2. What the surveys told us

Tables 18 and 19 show who the service providers were in nursing and home support/homemaking during the CCACs' four first years of existence (1996-2000). Tables 20 and 21 show the service providers in the areas of therapies and medical supplies/equipment for 1996-1999. A few words of caution: the tables do not tell us the value of the work to each provider agency, only that they received at least one contract with a CCAC. Moreover, it is possible for an agency to have had several contracts with a CCAC (e.g., for general nursing, pediatric nursing, and palliative care). However, it would only show up as being under contract once with that CCAC. So the tables show the number of CCACs in which an agency had contracts, not the number of contracts an agency had won in all. It should also be pointed out that not every provider agency will necessarily have shown up in the table, since not every CCAC responded.

The survey results are thus limited but they at least provide an initial portrait of home care in Ontario, however incomplete, during the

Table 18
Provider agencies under contract with CCACs, nursing, 1996-2000

1996-1997 (19 CCACs reporting)		1997-1998 (24 CCACs reporting)		1998-1999 (25 CCACs reporting)		1999-2000 (16 CCACs reporting)	
Victorian Order of Nurses	18	Victorian Order of Nurses	22	Victorian Order of Nurses	23	Victorian Order of Nurses	11
Para-Med Health Services	11	Para-Med Health Services	16	Para-Med Health Services	19	Para-Med Health Services	9
Comcare	10	Comcare	14	Comcare	15	Comcare	8
Saint Elizabeth Health Care	6	Saint Elizabeth Health Care	11	Saint Elizabeth Health Care	13	Saint-Elizabeth Health Care	7
Olsten Health Services	3	Olsten Health Services	6	Olsten Health Services	8	Olsten (Gentiva)	2
Bayshore Health (formerly Interim)	3	Bayshore Health (formerly Interim)	4	Bayshore Health (formerly Interim)	4	Bayshore Health	3
Special Care People (later Care Givers)	2	Special Care People (later Care Givers)	4	Special Care People (later Care Givers)	4	Care Givers	2
20 other public, private for-profit, and non-profit agencies, mostly under contract in only one locality.		21 other public, private for-profit, and non-profit agencies, mostly under contract in only one locality.		21 other public, private for-profit, and non-profit agencies, mostly under contract in only one locality.		13 other agencies, mostly under contract in only one locality	
27 agencies		27 agencies		28 agencies		20 agencies	

transition period to managed competition. They provide a benchmark against which to measure the results of the competitive process in full swing in much of Ontario home care since 1999. At the very least, they tell us who the main players are.

In establishing this list, we expected to find certain things. For example, because a large, albeit decreasing, volume of home care services was protected from competition between 1996 and 1999, we expected that the service providers most prevalent before managed competition would continue to show a strong presence during those years. Secondly, because the provincial government had directed CCACs (wherever possible) not to award the entire contract in each area to only one agency, we also expected that a number of agencies would begin to show up in places they had not previously been. Since the Victorian Order of Nurses and the Red Cross had respectively dominated the fields of visiting nursing and home support, we were not surprised to find them still present in most locations. The question was: of the others, which would expand and which would not?

In the field of nursing, our survey established a list of 28 service providers (see Table 18). Of these, there appear to be four dominant ones: the Victorian Order of Nurses, Para-Med Health Services, Comcare and Saint-Elizabeth Health Care. It is scarcely surprising to find the Victorian Order of Nurses among this group, since it was the provider of choice of visiting nursing services in home care prior to managed competition. The real question in its case is whether it has

Table 19
Provider agencies under contract with CCACs,
home support/homemaking, 1996-2000

1996-1997 (20 CCACs)		1997-1998 (23 CCACs)		1998-1999 (24 CCACs)		1999-2000 (16 CCACs)	
Red Cross	16	Red Cross	18	Red Cross	19	Red Cross	10
Para-Med	14	Para-Med	17	Para-Med	19	Para-Med	12
Comcare	12	Comcare	13	Comcare	13	Comcare	7
Olsten	6	Olsten	11	Olsten	10	Olsten (Gentiva)	6
Bayshore (Interim)	4	Bayshore (Interim)	7	Bayshore (Interim)	7	Bayshore	6
Victorian Order of Nurses	3	Victorian Order of Nurses	5	Victorian Order of Nurses	5	Victorian Order of Nurses	3
Saint-Elizabeth	3	Saint-Elizabeth	3	Saint-Elizabeth	6	Saint-Elizabeth	4
Med+ Care	3	Med+ Care	3	Med+ Care	3	Med+ Care	2
Central Health Services	2	Central Health Services	3	Central Health Services	3	Central Health Services	3
Spectrum	2	Spectrum	3	Spectrum	3	Spectrum	1
VHA	2	VHA	3	VHA	3	VHA	4
Two other agencies under contract in two localities and 42 other agencies under contract in only one locality.		12 other agencies under contract in 2 localities.		S.R.T. Med-Staff	3	S.R.T. Med-Staff	2
				Bradson	3	Bradson	3
		27 other agencies under contract in only one locality.		15 other agencies under contract in 2 localities.		7 other agencies under contract in 2 localities.	
				23 other agencies under contract in only one locality.		18 other agencies under contract in only one locality.	
55 agencies		50 agencies		51 agencies		39 agencies	

lost ground or not. Although the figures in the survey do not allow such a conclusion to be drawn, other sources indicate that it has been hurt by the managed competition process, as we have seen.

Of the other agencies, between 1996 and 1999, Saint-Elizabeth Health Care and Olsten appear to have more than doubled the number of locations in which they were present, while Para-Med Health Services nearly doubled its number of contracts too. Finally, Comcare also improved its share. While the first of the four is an old, established non-profit, with roots in the Catholic Church, the other three are the largest for-profit firms in the business in Ontario (see the section above profiling the provider agencies).

In our April 2000 survey, 16 CCACs responded, reporting a total of 20 agencies under contract in 1999-2000. The Victorian Order of Nurses was present in 11 of the locations, Para-Med in 9, Comcare in 8 and Saint-Elizabeth Health Care in 7, Olsten in 2. Given the number of responses, it would be risky to attempt to discern any trends in these numbers.

It is important to note that the fact that these agencies were under contract tells us nothing about the volume of service they were providing, nor does it indicate whether they were winning contracts in the RFP process or still receiving a protected share.

In home support and homemaking, the story in 1996-1999 was not dissimilar (see Table 19), although there is a less clearly defined dominant group. As expected, the survey shows the Red Cross present in most locations. More interestingly and significantly, of the more than fifty agencies under contract with the two dozen CCACs that responded, two agencies led the field in 1996-1999 along with the Red Cross, namely Para-Med and Comcare, with Olsten, Bayshore, the VON and Saint-Elizabeth Health Care also all steadily expanding over the three years. (It should be noted that a very large proportion of the agencies listed as being present in only one locality are in the Toronto area. A complete list of these can be found in the annual reports of the Toronto CCAC.)

Our April 2000 survey had 16 CCACs reporting a total of 39 agencies under contract. Para-Med was present in more locations than the Red Cross here (12 locations versus 10). Comcare appeared in 7, Bayshore Health Services in 6, the Visiting Homemakers' Association and Saint-Elizabeth Health Care in 4, Bradson Home Health Care, the VON and Central Health Services in 3. Again, we cannot make inferences from such small numbers.

In the fields of physiotherapy, occupational therapy, speech pathology, social work, and nutritional counselling, the majority of CCACs in 1998-1999 still provided services directly through their own in-house staff or through individual consultants hired on a fee-for-service basis. Throughout the three years, CCACs contracted with a significant number of outside agencies as well to offer various therapy services. In fact the number of such agencies increased with each year: 27 in 1996-1997, 44 in 1997-1998, and 53 in 1998-1999. Most were local social service agencies, hospitals and private clinics. We did not have sufficient data for 1999-2000 to warrant reporting it (see Table 20).

Finally, Table 21 lists some of the companies that sell medical supplies and equipment directly to CCACs. Many are local businesses, such as pharmacies. Others are part of larger chains, such as Shoppers Drug Mart, while others still are multinational corporations, such as Siemens, Hoechst Roussel, MDS, or Procter & Gamble. Note that half of the CCACs responding to the survey received supplies and equipment from local hospitals.

Table 20
Provider agencies under contract with CCACs,
physiotheraphy, speech pathology & social work, 1996-1999

1996-1997 (19 CCACs)		1997-1998 (24 CCACs)		1998-1999 (25 CCACs)	
In-house staff/fee-for-service consultants	11	In-house staff/fee-for-service consultants	15	In-house staff/fee-for-service consultants	14
Para-Med	3	Para-Med	6	Para-Med	5
Comcare	2	Comcare	5	Comcare	5
Community Rehab	2	Community Rehab	3	Community Rehab	3
				Communicare	3
3 other agencies supplying services in two localities, and 21 other agencies and hospitals supplying services in one locality.		5 other agencies supplying services in two localities, and 36 other agencies and hospitals supplying services in only one locality.		9 other agencies supplying services in two localities, and 38 other agencies and hospitals supplying services in only one locality.	

Table 21
Provider agencies under contract with CCACs, equipment and medical supplies, 1996-1999

1996-1997 (12 CCACs)		1997-1998 (15 CCACs)		1998-1999 (17 CCACs)	
Shoppers Home Health Care/Doncaster	7	Shoppers Home Health Care/Doncaster	7	Shoppers Home Health Care/Doncaster	8
Therapy Supplies	4	Therapy Supplies	6	Therapy Supplies	8
Caremark	4	Caremark	7	Caremark	7
Miscellaneous Hospitals	7	Miscellaneous Hospitals	7	Miscellaneous Hospitals	5
Medigas	3	Medigas	4	Medigas	6
KCI Medical	3	KCI Medical	3	KCI Medical	3
Starkman Surgical	2	Starkman Surgical	3	Starkman Surgical	3
Baxter	2	Baxter	2	Baxter	2
Ingram & Bell	2	Ingram & Bell	2	Ingram & Bell	2
Red Cross	2	Red Cross	1	Red Cross	1
Smith & Nephew	2	Smith & Nephew	1	Smith & Nephew	1
				Respircare	4
28 other companies that supply equipment and supplies to only one CCAC.		24 other companies that supply equipment and supplies to only one CCAC.		21 other companies that supply equipment and supplies to only one CCAC.	

To sum up, our surveys suggest that between 1996 and 1999, a handful of mostly for-profit agencies expanded significantly across Ontario, in the area of nursing, home support and therapy services. Because part of the total volume of service was protected until 1999, some of the contracts included in the 1996-1999 data were won in the RFP process and some were not. It is only in the contracts awarded from 1999 on that we shall be able to get a clear picture of non-profit agencies' ability to compete successfully with for-profits in the managed competition process. Unfortunately, we have too little information at this point to be able to form such a clear picture.

3. What the surveys did not tell us

During 1996-1999, only a portion of the nursing contracts were allocated through the managed competition process; most of the service was still awarded on a non-competitive basis. The survey does not tell us which agency won contracts under the protected share, which won under competition, and what the distribution was among agencies. The figures in Tables 6 to 9 *tell us nothing about the volume of service awarded each agency in each of the three years.* An agency could show up as still being under contract, but be receiving far less work than before. The information in Tables 6 to 9 is therefore *incomplete*.

This is a very important point: *it may be that agencies maintain their rank in the table, even while losing some of their volume of service.* Non-profits may have continued to be present in many of the same locations during 1996-1999, but have lost some of their volume to the for-profits.

In our August-September 1999 survey, we asked the CCACs to identify the share of contracts going to non-profit and for-profit agencies respectively. In retrospect, our results are unclear because we are not sure how the question was interpreted. Did the respondents understand the question to refer to the *number* of contracts awarded, to the *total dollar value* of the contracts, or to the volume of service awarded (i.e. number of professional visits and homemaking hours). Nonetheless, the results indicate a growing presence of for-profits in the delivery of home care services. In the survey, 13 percent of CCACs reported an increase in the percentage of contracts going to non-profit agencies, 57 percent reported an increase in the percentage of contracts going to for-profit agencies, and 30 percent reported no change in the distribution of contracts between non-profit and for-profit agencies. Overall, CCACs reported in the fall of 1999 that less than 1 percent of contracts go to public-sector agencies (e.g., hospitals), 47 percent go to non-profit agencies, and 53 percent go to for-profit agencies. The formulation of the question did not allow the different service areas (nursing, home support/homemaking, therapies, supplies/equipment) to be disaggregated.

We did ask CCACs in our December 1999/January 2000 survey to indicate the share of service volume going respectively to non-profits and for-profits in each of the four major expenditure areas (nursing, home support, therapies, supplies/equipment). Unfortunately, the response rate on this issue was low: 14 out of 43 CCACs. Furthermore, only half of the 14 respondents provided statistics for 1996-1997 and 1997-1998. We simply do not have enough information to form any meaningful picture of what is going on as yet. More research is needed.

What more do we need to find out?

To conclude this section, it is too soon to say who will ultimately win the most contracts and the greatest volume of work. Competitive bidding was introduced only gradually and is not yet in effect everywhere. One CCAC will still have its own in-house staff providing homemaking and home support until October 2000, for example. Some have tendered therapy services, only to find that none of the bids were adequate. Others have found that the volume of work is too small for it to be feasible to tender it.

The figures we were able to gather are too incomplete to be the basis of any strong conclusions. In does appear that for-profits are gaining ground on non-profits. Time will tell whether this will continue or whether the non-profits will reassert or affirm their predominance in their areas of traditional strength.

However, who wins the contracts is only part of the story. Equally important is *how they win them, how they have to change in order to be successful.*

How non-profit agencies have adapted to the new competitive environment

When asked what difference there was between non-profit and for-profit provider agencies, one CCAC manager told me that there was none on the front line. Another CCAC manager expressed frustration at hearing criticism of the shift from non-profit to for-profit providers. He said that the selection process was entirely fair and was based strictly on the quality of the bids, not on some being cheaper than others. He also stressed that he found the for-profit agencies more efficient than the non-profits, referring specifically to issues such as billing and following up on complaints.

What do such comments signify? On the one hand, common sense and experience indicate that there are good and bad, efficient and inefficient, non-profit and for-profit agencies. No amount of general arguments demonstrating the superiority of non-profit provision allows us to deduce that, consequently, each and every specific non-profit will be superior to each and every for-profit. By the same rules of logic, the existence of such examples of course does not in any way invalidate the general arguments.

But there is more. On what basis are the non-profits and for-profits now judged? For example, the administrative superiority of one agency may mean that it investigates and addresses complaints more swiftly than another. But this is not in itself an indicator of the professionalism of the front-line nurses and other care workers, or of the quality of the care they provide.

On the other hand, how should we read the other manager's comment that there is no difference on the front line? Should we see it as a reflection of the specific conditions in that area? Is it a tribute to the professionalism of nurses and other care-giving staff throughout the system? Does the comment tell us that the whole system is set up in such a way that the CCAC managers are not really in a position to see what is going on at the front line? Was there never a difference in the past, or is it rather the case that non-profit agencies have grown increasingly similar to their for-profit rivals as they have had to adapt to the new competitive environment? Unfortunately, such questions cannot be answered without in-depth studies of the conditions prevailing in a representative sample of CCACs, an impossible undertaking in the context of this study.

We do know, however, that the new competitive environment did begin to take its toll on some of the non-profit agencies by 1998. Even where they won contracts, they had to adapt to the new competitive environment by adopting many market-determined norms of efficiency. This meant diversifying their operations, like for-profit firms, for example by aggressively pursuing homemaking contracts; cutting costs; restructuring management; changing the work process; and sometimes downgrading working conditions.

Non-profit organizations appear to have started out with a number of handicaps. As registered charities, they are compelled by Revenue Canada to divulge key financial information about their operations. Some have felt that this placed them at a disadvantage in relation to for-profit companies, which are under no such obligation, and could use the information about the charities to undercut their bids.[106]

In head-to-head competition with for-profit firms, non-profits such as the Victorian Order of Nurses (VON) were clearly at a disadvantage with respect to costs. Non-profit agencies are covered by pay-equity legislation, while at least some for-profit firms are not.[107] Some CCACs have established ceilings of $17.75 an hour for home-care contracts; yet non-profit agencies are mandated by law to charge a rate of $16.60 an hour for their workers. This leaves hardly any room for administration costs. Unconstrained by pay-equity laws, for-profit firms can put in bids $2 to $3 an hour lower. Non-profits thus have the deck stacked against them.[108] There are also fears that firms may deliberately submit very low bids, "loss leaders" in the language of the retail trade, in an effort to undercut the competition and drive it out of business.[109]

The Victorian Order of Nurses has had a unionized workforce for several years, and has tended to hire its employees on a full-time, regular basis. Many for-profit firms, by contrast, have tended to offer their employees part-time or casual positions. In a competitive market where nurses are in short supply, this could play in favour of the VON, because it could attract scarce nurses through its higher wages.[110] On the other hand, hospitals and long-term care facilities pay higher wages than home care agencies. As a CCAC CEO put it:

> I am worried about the effect that has on our ability to attract and retain people in care in the community. We get in a homemaker and provide their personal-support-worker training, then long-term-care facilities pay more money and we lose them to that sector. Nurses come to work in the community, then as soon as hospitals have an opening, they go to work in the hospital, which pays more. There are some serious human resource issues across the province, perhaps across the nation. As long as care in the community is paid less than in hospitals, we'll have a problem, and as long as we're in a competitive environment, it's going to be hard to get those costs up.[111]

In the face of competition, non-profits have changed their organizational structures. They have eliminated managerial positions, increasing workloads, and cut costs, for example by replacing full-time permanent positions with part-time temporary ones; paying nurses on a piece-work basis (i.e., per visit); holding the line on pay increases and cutting benefits; reducing or doing away with nursing team meetings, orientation and continuing education[112]; increasing the time nurses can spend away from the office, for example through increased use of voice mail, pagers and cellular telephones; and last, but not least, transforming the work of registered nurses by downloading aspects of their work to less qualified workers.

The director of a non-profit provider agency told me that nurses are saying that clients are sicker. The nurses are concentrating on IVs, complex dressing changes and the like. They are leaving many tasks to other, less-skilled, providers if the latter can do them as well. Nurses are seeing more people and getting more high-tech. In the process, it would appear that their work is becoming more clinical in nature, and that there may be less time for the social dimension of care. Just as in acute-care settings, where total quality management has cut out much of the time nurses could spend with the patient,[113] so in the "hospital at home" nurses must concentrate on specific technical tasks and have less time for the more holistic practice of caring for the individual as a whole person.[114]

Paying nurses on a piecework basis enables agencies to keep their wage bills down. "When a visit that was supposed to take 1 hour now takes 1.5 hours, because of the increased complexity, the nurse effectively faces a lower hourly wage. (....) Increasingly, nurses also report significant pressure from employers to see more clients in less time. This is the result of financial incentives created by the fee-for-service approach and the absence of system monitoring of patient outcomes."[115] Piecework creates the incentive for nurses to visit more clients and to shorten each visit in order to fit more visits into each day—an incentive obviously at odds with the quality of care, which ought obviously to be the only concern.

Agencies used to be able to balance out high-volume/low-cost visits and low-volume/high-cost ones. But with more and more very ill service users, this has become more difficult. Nurses are being required to spend the same time with users, despite their increasing needs and the growing complexity of nursing tasks. As in hospitals, it would seem that there may be a trend in home care to assign tasks to "generic workers" instead of nurses. This is particularly dramatic in a sector where workers must show up for work in the service-user's home on time and must perform their duties with virtually no supervision in a range of difficult and sometimes dangerous circumstances.[116] "For high-quality home care services to be delivered to clients, workers must have the capacity to act independently, travel extensively to serve their clients, and solve problems which are unique to the physical and social environment of the home setting." They also must be able to form a good working relationship with clients and clients' families. Home care requires "a complex set of interpersonal, communication, administrative skills and knowledge."[117]

Pressured by the competitive environment, agencies have squeezed their employees' wages and benefits. In negotiations between the Victorian Order of Nurses and the Practical Nurses' Federation of Ontario, the agency's management proposed eliminating the travel subsidy which reimbursed nurses' very considerable travel expenses at a rate of 26 to 30 cents per kilometre (which meant $11,000 per year for some nurses).[118] Susan Coke, Executive Director of the VON's Ottawa-Carleton branch, was quoted as saying that her agency "needed the savings to compete against for-profit home-care businesses after the market was opened to competition by Ontario's conservative government."[119] Accusing the VON of trying to resolve its budgetary problems at their expense, hundreds of registered practical nurses went on strike. In September 1998, it was the turn of registered nurses belonging to the Ontario Nurses Association to be confronted with the same demand and to strike as well.[120]

In a further development, the Windsor branch of the Red Cross announced that it would close after 53 years of activity in the community. In August 1999, the Red Cross asked its 196 homemakers, who must travel considerable distances annually to get to and from clients' homes, to accept a 50-percent cut in their travel allowance. However, before the union had had a chance to vote on the proposal, the Red Cross submitted a bid to the Windsor-Essex CCAC for the homemaking contract, and based the bid on the lower travel allowance which had not yet been accepted by the workers. In an internal memo quoted in *The Windsor Star*, Red Cross management told the workers that "to remain competitive and be successful in continuing to receive work from the CCAC, Red Cross submitted their bid based on a lower travel allowance rate (...) If the union does not accept the reduction, we will be forced to close the Windsor-Essex Homemaker Service."[121] When the workers did in fact vote against the proposed cut, the Red Cross announced it would close the branch and lay off all the employees.[122]

The executive director of one non-profit agency told me that competition was good, because it compelled agencies to be efficient and innovative. At the same time, she deplored the disparities in salaries, and the fact that for-profit firms hire their staff on temporary, part-time contracts with no, or fewer benefits, something she considers the outcome of privatization.[123] It is hard to have it both ways: market competition and poorer working conditions are linked. The whole point of competition is that the threat of losing contracts and potentially going under supposedly spurs organizations to be "efficient." That very threat also encourages organizations to pay lower wages and benefits, and to hire their staff on a temporary, part-time basis. By their very nature, for-profit firms are always driven by the search for higher profits and are therefore perpetually interested in offering their employees the lowest possible compensation. Non-profit agencies, by contrast, must break even over time, but are not constrained by the same imperative to accumulate profits. Yet, they too may be pushed in that direction in a competitive environment, as the non-profit agency's executive director agreed.

Lower costs—for now

Not surprisingly, in the light of this, the immediate result of managed competition seems to have been a decline in the cost of care, which was no doubt the effect sought after by the government:

> Nurses have reported that the unit price of delivering care has dropped with the implementation of the RFP process. In the first round of competition (for short-term contracts) prices were from 3 to 13 percent lower ($3-4 less per visit), equivalent to 1992 rates. More recently, prices for longer-term contracts appear to be stabilizing at 1995-1996 levels. It is critical to note that this initial drop and subsequent stabilization has occurred at the same time as the volume and complexity of care required in the community has increased dramatically.[124]

The CEO of one CCAC noted that all the bidders it dealt with were nervous the first year and submitted bids that were low:

> We probably saved a million dollars that first year. In the second year, all the prices went up [...] and consistently so across the board—and at that the cost is probably still too low. People in community care are paid too little. Homemakers and nurses are not paid enough in my mind. Even though we say that quality is the driver, because cost only weighs 10 percent in our scheme, when companies bid for contracts they still believe that cost is a big player and would not risk putting in a very elevated cost.[125]

But it is not clear that managed competition is always the cheaper option. Free-market apologists hold that the private sector is always cheaper and more efficient than the public sector, but this is far from always true in the real world. In the case of CCACs, this is illustrated by the enforced divestment of therapists. The Ottawa-Carleton CCAC found that divestment would cost it half a million dollars more than simply continuing to provide the service itself.[126] Rather than tell the CCAC not to divest itself of the service, the province said it would be willing to let the CCAC retain a potential year-end surplus of half a million dollars to cover the extra cost. It also declared that it would "consider as an allowable cost one-time funding to cover the payment of specific severance costs incurred by the successful employer who takes over the employment of direct service workers and subsequently must lay off these workers as a result of failure to maintain a sufficient level of business as a result of loss of a Request for Proposals in the Ottawa-Carleton area."[127] In other words, were the firm which won the bid to deliver the therapeutic services divested by the CCAC to lose the contract in the following bidding round, the province would allow the CCAC to pay the severance pay of the workers that the firm would then lay off. Not only, then, did the province's plan cost the CCAC more money at the moment of divestment, it may also cost the CCAC again should the successor company fail to have its contract renewed. It is likely too that administrative costs are much higher under managed competition than they would be in a strictly public system.

Finally, as an executive with a provider agency told me, "I am absolutely convinced that the average cost will go up significantly in the next three to five years." Prices have diminished in the short term, but it is likely that they will go up significantly, and even higher than ever before. Provider agencies used to be able to take advantages of economies of scale to keep their unit prices steady over the years, while breaking even by receiving an increasing volume of work. But with the new segmented markets for nursing, homemaking, and so on, average costs will go up. Moreover, there is a very real shortage of staff now. If home care is to recruit the nurses it will need, salaries, benefits, and working conditions will have to improve, and that will drive up prices. If that is true, managed competition will have achieved the opposite of what it was intended to do.

Conclusion

One of the outcomes of rising home care expenditures is new business opportunities for private industry—an attractive prospect in the eyes of a governing party with the motto "Open for Business," and a government which has made public its interest in divesting itself of its service delivery functions through contracting out, private-public partnerships and the like. It is also not impossible that those very business interests have lobbied the government to bring about the changes in question.

Several individuals interviewed in the course of this study expressed doubt that much money could be made in home care. This may be truer of a labour-intensive product-line such as homemaking, where profitability is based on volume and market share is all-important, where employees paid $9.65 an hour or a few pennies more move from agency to agency, and there is little to distinguish one from another. Yet, the National Forum on Health pointed out in its final report that *"the private sector is pressing to gain access to new business opportunities in a sector that, up to now, has been beyond its reach."*[128] This is scarcely surprising, given the sustained steep rise in public investment in home care for the past twenty years. Furthermore, to dominate a sector of industry, it is not necessary for firms to own all the enterprises in it; it is enough to control *strategic points*, from which profits may be siphoned off. In the contemporary economy, these are typically the production of management systems and new technologies. It is not surprising then to see that for-profit companies have by and large been the purveyors of medical supplies and equipment to home care agencies (although public hospitals have contributed as well). Now, as those agencies revamp their management structures and systems, as they adopt new technologies, there are new opportunities for firms with expertise in those areas (including some of the agencies themselves, potentially) to gain new markets or increased market share.[129] It should be remembered too that a growing share—forty percent or more—of home-care users are acute-care patients discharged from hospitals.[130] If treatment of these patients is a much more high-tech affair, it should not be surprising to see for-profit firms taking over the more capital-intensive end of the home-care market. Offering homemaking services is part of such a context; it has to do with product diversification and offering a full range of services.

Market competition supposedly lowers costs, improves efficiency, enhances quality, and increases the variety and quantity of services. Yet, while it has driven agencies to lower their costs in the short run, it will likely have the opposite effect in the longer run. It has led to a process of redefining efficiency and quality which will make them more measurable, but erodes the networks of trust which are the basis for true quality and effectiveness. The attraction of the competitive bidding model is the great hope that it will lead to standardized quality indicators and reporting methods across Ontario, thus making it possible to hold workers, agencies and CCACs themselves accountable to the Ministry of Health and Long-Term Care for their use of tax dollars. Yet, it will also erode the continuity of care—thus showing a lack of accountability to the people who actually need and use the services.

The balance in home care is tipping from public to private payers, from non-profit to for-profit providers, but also from paid to unpaid workers.

1. An ever greater share of care and dollars is moving from hospital care, the sector covered by the Canada Health Act, to home care, which (a) is not covered by the Canada Health Act, and (b) now features a system of managed competition in which for-profit service providers are winning an increasing share of the work.
2. Publicly funded home care is rationed and it is necessary for many of those receiving care to pay for it out-of-pocket or by way of private insurance; for many others, it is necessary to do without, to rely on the informal care of friends, family and neighbours, or to be institutionalized in a retirement residence or other facility, most of which are private, for-profit enterprises, and in which standards are, to say the least, uneven.
3. What information we have been able to collect shows that managed competition has enabled for-profit agencies to build their presence in the sector. Furthermore, managed competition is also putting pressure on non-profits to adopt some of the management structures, systems and strategies of for-profit businesses in order to survive (e.g., cutting employees' wages and benefits, curtailing services, etc.). Even if non-profit providers succeed in not being supplanted by the for-profits, what will it cost them, their workers and the people they serve, to survive in the new market environment?
4. As non-profits' management strategies and operational structure comes more and more to resemble that of for-profit companies under the influence of the competitive process, it is not inconceivable that for-profit companies might in the future seek to buy out the assets and home care operations of non-profit agencies in order to secure a monopoly, as they have done in other sectors of industry.

Managed competition and private for-profit provision are clearly at the heart of the provincial government's agenda, a government committed to replacing public governance, oversight and control through democratic and community institutions, by private ownership and control through the market.

Conclusion

Medicare has worked well for Canadians. They identify with it and believe in it. They are concerned about its future. And yet, despite this popular support, they keep being told that the system is not working and needs restructuring and privatization.

I argued in these pages that privatization is a *process* with a specific
- *content* (the dismantling of welfare state social protection, or re-commodification, and the loss of social rights);
- *structure* ("cascading privatization");
- and *ideological form* ("reinventing government," "patient-centered care," "community").

These three elements work together in various ways at various levels and at various periods. Federal preoccupations and policies lead to cutbacks and commercialization. The loss of a portion of federal transfers encourages the provinces to accelerate their own cutbacks and processes of restructuring, commercializing, contracting out, and privatizing public services. In the name of doing better with less, of bringing government closer to the people, of easing the tax burden, of focusing on the patient, governments implement market-style reforms of public administration. Hospitals, the main institutions at the receiving end of government cutbacks and restructuring directives in health care, then speed up their own adoption of private-sector re-engineering strategies and shed many of their functions and activities, as well as passing more and more of their patients on to other health-care institutions, such as long-term care facilities and home care agencies. Many individuals simply end up at home sick without care. How many people live in fear of being ill and being refused admission to the hospital or being sent home too soon?

Restructuring is driven by bureaucratic concerns with cost-containment at the federal, provincial and local levels. It is also the result of the technocratic project of re-engineering health-care delivery systems to enhance their "efficiency," and make them conform to higher "standards." It is falsely presented as the appropriate response to grassroots complaints about lack of access, lack of control and lack of transparency.

Yet these processes, partly by creating such a sense of crisis and partly by being the wrong answers to the real issues, breed discontent and a desire for reform. Although Canadians firmly believe in medicare, how long will it be before they begin to fall prey to the false promise that private health-care markets or for-profit health care delivery will solve all the problems?

Underlying restructuring and privatization in their many facets, though, are the same business-oriented political forces and the same market ideology. Every level of government and all the major health care institutions are part of networks that include large corporations, multinational consulting firms, and Canadian and foreign think tanks. These central policy organs of the privatization drive are the Adam Smith Institute in the UK, the Heritage Foundation and Reason Foundation in the United States, and the Fraser Institute in Canada. But there are also international organizations peddling the same message, such as the Organization for Economic Co-operation and Development (OECD), the World Bank, and the International Monetary Fund. According to Brendan Martin, there are six large consulting firms promoting privatization world wide: Ernst & Young, Coopers & Lybrand Deloitte, DRT International, Price Waterhouse, Arthur Andersen, KPMG Peat Marwick.[1] These are the very companies that hospitals and other institutions in Ontario turn to when they seek advice on restructuring.

The big transnational accountancy firms developed their public sector consultancy arms largely by doing studies in such matters as "value for money" and "efficiency" for governments and municipalities, as concern about costs, structures and organizational methods grew in the late 1970s and early 1980s. (Indeed, they are still doing plenty such work. For example, in Canada, DRT were handed contracts worth more than $2 million in 1991 to carry out "operational reviews" of two federal government departments; Price Waterhouse were awarded contracts worth nearly Canadian $1 million to do the same in two other departments; and Peat Marwick were paid more than Canadian $750,000 to look at the workings of the country's Public Service Commission.) So they helped to develop the climate of commercialization in which service design is increasingly cost-led. Privatization in various forms followed, in a climate in which the ability of firms to cut costs came to be regarded as more important than their suitability to carry out the service.[2]

Faced with rising social costs, diminishing tax revenues, soaring interest rates and swelling deficits, governments in the 1980s sought advice from international institutions, bankers, consulting firms and think tanks, and received the same verdict everywhere: reduce government spending, slash social programs, commercialize, contract out and privatize government services, let the market regulate and provide. Institutions such as hospitals went to the same consultants and received the same advice.

It is true that health care restructuring did not at first take the form of privatization, but of *corporate rationalization*.[3] The theme of corporate rationalization extends throughout this study; it is surely a key trend in the recent evolution of the health care system in Ontario, indeed in Canada and other countries. *Privatization* in Ontario's health care system has remained marginal, *if* by privatization one means the outright sale of publicly-owned enterprises, the widespread introduction of user fees, or the wholesale transfer of governance, service delivery and financing to the private sector. In this sense, a recent article in the Medical Reform Group's newsletter suggested, "frank large-scale privatization is unlikely to occur in the near future."[4]

However, *privatization is not marginal if we consider its more subtle manifestations*. Pat Armstrong and others have talked about "privatization by stealth" and "creeping privatization" in the case of health care in Ontario.[5] Changes are occurring, some of which, taken singly, may seem peripheral. Yet, when looked at in their totality, they signal much greater changes that may come. I have already recalled the Mulroney government's "social policy by stealth"—a policy of quietly making many unheralded and unpublicized changes in tax and social policy. That "stealthy" approach set the stage for the very massive changes in social policy brought about by the Chrétien government.

It may be that Ontario is on the verge of seeing such developments. Given the enormous popularity and prestige of Canadian medicare, no government could introduce privatization rapidly. The bitter and widespread opposition to the Alberta government's Bill 11, which will allow district health authorities to contract out some surgical procedures requiring in-patient stays to for-profit hospitals, provides a good illustration of this. Medicare is the last redoubt of the welfare state in Canada. Every other institution has been challenged, hollowed out or dismantled over the past fifteen years.

But those changes did not all come at once. It was first necessary for the federal and provincial governments, business lobbyists and others to wage a multi-year campaign to convince Canadians of the indispensability of reform. This campaign took several forms. Canadians were overwhelmed over many years by rhetoric about the country's fiscal crisis and the need for restraint. They were also constantly told that the social programs of the past could no longer be sustained in the face of the competitive pressures of the new global economy. The gradual deterioration of those social programs after years of cutbacks also gradually eroded public support. The battle over medicare is under way: doom-filled predictions of its looming fiscal crisis are rife in the media; sensational accounts of the inefficiency or impotence of public health care facilities (e.g., hospital emergency wards) are legion.

Arguments in favour of a greater private-sector presence are proliferating. Proposals to privatize the cost of health care that have long since been refuted and discredited from a strictly intellectual standpoint—what health economist Robert Evans calls "zombies"—once again stalk the land.[6]

The stage is set for the middle classes to begin deserting the medicare ship and climbing onto the "lifeboats" of private insurance and private providers. Little do they know, many of them will be cast out of the lifeboats, as insurance premiums go up and coverage proves less comprehensive than they might have thought.

Alberta's policy of allowing for-profit hospitals will lock not only all future Alberta governments, but potentially all other provincial governments, into having to deal with for-profit corporations in the hospital sector, under the provisions of the North American Free Trade Agreement:

> if the Klein government allows for-profit hospitals, the law will bind every succeeding Alberta government. Despite Premier Klein's assertions that this policy can be tried out like a new suit, a future Alberta government that wished to terminate the experiment with for-profit care would be faced with a major problem. While the legislature still could pass any law that it wished, any company (either one which did not have its contract renewed or one which was not even part of the original market) could sue the Alberta government for expropriation of its assets.[7]

Ontario has not moved to create new private hospitals. But it has introduced managed competition in home care, ambulance services, and other areas. This raises the question as to whether any future Ontario government could rescind managed competition and establish a public-sector or exclusively not-for-profit delivery system in those areas.

Prominent economists have made the case that for-profit medicine is more expensive, less efficient and less equitable. Major studies in the United States (notably articles that appeared in the *New England Journal of Medicine* between 1997 and 1999) have indicated that not-for-profit health care is cheaper and more efficient, and led to much better health outcomes than its for-profit competitors.[8] Studies in Canada have yielded similar results, showing for example that waiting lists for cataract surgery are longer in private than in public hospitals, and that care is cheaper in the latter than in the former.[9]

If publicly funded and provided health care is cheaper, more efficient, and leads to fewer deaths and better health, why on earth would anyone want to privatize it? It has even been suggested that medicare offers business a source of comparative advantage over the United States, because it is considerably cheaper than private insurance.[10] The answer clearly lies both in the profits to be made and in the struggle over the distribution of wealth in society.

Robert Evans has pointed out that medicare is a social program that redistributes wealth from the wealthy and healthy to the "unwealthy" and unhealthy. A single-payer system based on income tax, such as exists in Ontario, will require the wealthy to pay proportionately more as long as the income tax remains progressive. A system based on user charges would hurt the "unwealthy" and benefit the wealthy, because such charges are a very regressive form of taxation. Private *producers*, e.g. drug companies, are opposed to a single-payer, income-tax based system and favour the user charge/private insurance model, precisely because the former would reduce the overall cost of drugs, i.e. would eat into corporate profits.

As Evans points out, it is not clear that any of the proponents of privatization really want a *totally* private system. The public system is much too bountiful as a potential cash cow for private corporations. The aim is rather to limit the public system in various ways, so as to maximize the opportunities for profit in its margins, interstices and gaps:

> It is not clear how many, if any, of these would support a *truly* private system, with no direct or indirect contribution of public funds. (...) The economic mayhem among providers would be truly awesome. Instead what seems to be contemplated is a continuation of public support on a large scale, but without limits on private fee setting or delivery, or private insurance—rather like the United States, in fact, before widespread "managed care."

(...) If governments continue to be effective at containing costs, growth in incomes must come from private revenue sources. But the objective is to increase the total flow of funds into health care, not merely to replace one source with another. Encourage fiscally pressed (or ideologically sympathetic) governments to shift their focus from containing overall system costs, to containing their own budgetary outlays. Just get rid of the associated restrictions on access to private funds, and let the total costs go where they will, i.e. where they should, i.e. where we want them to, i.e. up.[11]

This would offer scope for physicians and other private entrepreneurs to open private clinics funded through private insurance, especially if they could obtain public subsidies for the latter (e.g., as in tax breaks presently given for employer-funded dental and pharmaceutical plans). Physicians could then play both markets, continuing to see their patients in the publicly funded hospitals, while also seeing their other patients in private clinics. This appears to be the dynamic underpinning the private-hospital initiative in Alberta.

But it is not just about developing private sources of revenue to supplement money from public sources. It is also a matter of skimming off more of that public money, by moving into areas such as laboratory services, home care, ambulance services, and by developing new markets in public institutions for management systems, drugs, technology, and services, as has been happening in Ontario.

Today, government redistribution of the wealth flows from the unhealthy and "unwealthy" to the healthy and wealthy. And instead of initiating major investments to create new public assets, such as hospitals, the public sector itself has now become the booty of private corporations. In the "Superbuild Fund," for example, money that might in an earlier era have been used to create public goods will be channelled into the private sector to build, own, and operate services and physical assets such as roads, schools or hospitals, which private corporations will rent to the state or to private citizens by way of user charges.

Many corporations prefer today to buy out their competitors, rather than invest in new plant and workers.[12] Similarly, private companies are now poised to take over the ownership and delivery of strategic parts of the public health care system built up by the public sector, while still enjoying the manna of tax dollars flowing into their pockets.

Not to put too fine a point on it, the privatization of the health care system is a form of plunder by the private sector. In the post-war years, Canadian governments invested massive resources in building up public infrastructures, services and programs. These were the property of the state and therefore of all citizens. They constituted a portion of the national wealth; all citizens had—at least in principle—an entitlement to benefit from these public goods. Selling them off, charging user fees for their use, rationing them, closing them down, all represent a disentitlement of citizens, an expropriation of our common heritage.

In some ways, this is reminiscent of the enclosures movement that occurred in Britain between the 16th and the 19th centuries.[13] Extensive tracts of land had from medieval times been held in common for the use of villages or local communities. The common people had more or less extensive rights to the use of the land and to its fruits. As a result of the enclosures, the common people were stripped of these rights, the land was expropriated and fenced in, becoming a single large *private* holding. The people who had lived on the land and lived off its fruits were driven away.[14] They often became homeless vagabonds or cheap labour working for the new exclusive landlords, who most often turned use of the land over to sheep farming. Thomas More (the philosopher famous as the "man for all seasons") described this as "sheep devouring men."[15] As citizens of Ontario and Canada, we must remain vigilant, lest we be devoured by forces of which we are scarcely even aware.

Notes

Preface

1. See Robert Evans, "Health Reform: What 'Business' Is It of Business?" in Daniel Drache and Terry Sullivan (eds.), *Market Limits in Health Reform: Public Success, Private Failure*, London, Routledge, 1999, 31.
2. The values of universality, accessibility, comprehensiveness, portability, and public administration are the five national standards of health care enshrined in the Canada Health Act (1984). For a discussion, see the annual reports on provincial compliance with the Canada Health Act published by Health Canada.
3. As Colleen Fuller puts it: "The creation of Canada's medicare system was the result of a long struggle, countless compromises, and a rejection by many millions of people of what existed at the time, in favour of what could be." (Colleen Fuller, *Caring for Profit: How Corporations Are Taking Over Canada's Health Care System*, Vancouver, New Star Books/Ottawa, Canadian Centre for Policy Alternatives, 1998, 12.)
4. Quoted in Richard Mackie, "Most Ontarians believe health care deteriorating," *The Globe and Mail*, January 17, 2000.
5. See the town hall meeting with federal Finance Minister Paul Martin on CBC Newsworld, March 1, 2000, for an example of such expressions of anxiety.
6. See Ontario Premier Mike Harris's remarks leading up to the signing of the 1999 social union agreement and following the 2000 federal budget (*Ottawa Citizen*, March 1, 2000; *The Globe and Mail*, March 1, 2000).
7. Paul Starr, "The New Life of the Liberal State: Privatization and the Restructuring of State-Society Relations," in John Waterbury and Ezra Suleiman, eds., *Public Enterprise and Privatization*, Boulder, Westview Press, 1990; and Paul Starr, "The Meaning of Privatization," *Yale Law and Policy Review*, 6 (1988), 6-41.
8. "The label 'private' in the context of health care is being used in many different ways by different people for different purposes. The most basic distinction is between payment for and provision of health care services. The financing of health care may be drawn from public or from private sources: this is logically independent of whether the services themselves are provided by public or private agencies. But the distinctions on the provision side are not always as clear as on the financing side. At one end of the spectrum is provision of care by government employees working for government agencies. At the

other end are purely for-profit, publicly traded corporations, such as drug and equipment manufacturers and some providers of laboratory and long-term care services. Most health care is provided by not-for-profit and 'not-only-for-profit' organizations that respond to motivations and 'bottom lines' that are very different from those of for-profit corporations." (Robert G. Evans, Morris L. Barer, Steven Lewis, Michael Rachlis, Greg L. Stoddart, *Private Highway, One-Way Street: The Deklein and Fall of Canadian Medicare?* Vancouver, Health Policy Research Unit, Centre for Health Services and Policy Research, University of British Columbia, March 2000, Executive Summary, at http://www.chspr.ubc.ca>)

9 "It must be recognized that it is an oversimplification to classify a country's health system as either public or private. Virtually every country employs some combination of financing and delivery models, relying on various public-private combinations in various sectors of the health system or for various groups of the nation's population. (...) Similarly, the public and private sectors are involved to a lesser or greater extent in service delivery, depending on the health sector within which services are provided (e.g., dental, vision, rehabilitation, long-term care), on the population group for which services are geared (e.g., state employees, veterans, the elderly), or on the perceived urgency of the services (acute versus chronic care, elective versus urgent surgery)." (Raisa Deber, Lutchmie Narine, Pat Baranek, Natasha Sharpe, Katya Masnyk Duvalko, Randi Zlotnik-Shaul, Peter Coyte, George Pink, Paul Williams, *The Public-Private Mix in Health Care*, in *Striking a Balance: Health Care Systems in Canada and Elsewhere*, Canada Health Action: Building on the Legacy—Papers commissioned by the National Forum on Health, Volume 4, Sainte-Foy, Éditions Multimondes, 1998, 439-440.

10 The *or* is important here. I disagree with the too narrow definition proposed by Lundqvist: "the active and conscious transfer of responsibility from the public to the private realm, involving three main activities: regulation, financing, and production." (Lennart Lundqvist, "Privatization: Towards a Concept for Comparative Analysis," *Journal of Public Opinion*, 8:1, 1, quoted by S. D. VanderBent, *The Role and Value of the Private Sector in Home Health and Social Care Provision*, Position Paper, Ontario Home Health Care Providers Association, March 1999, 6-7.

11 Kevin Taft and Gillian Steward, *Clear Answers: The Economics and Politics of For-Profit Medicine*, Edmonton, Duval House Publishing/The University of Alberta Press/Parkland Institute, 2000, 22.

12 Quoted by April Lindgren, "Ontario open to ideas on privatization," *Ottawa Citizen*, February 10, 2000.

13 Richard Mackie, "Harris calls on Canadians to weigh in on health care," *The Globe and Mail*, February 14, 2000.
14 See Åke Blomqvist, "Introduction: Economic Issues in Canadian Health Care," and William G. Tholl, "Health Care Spending in Canada: Skating Faster on Thinner Ice,"in Åke Blomqvist and David M. Brown (eds.), *Limits to Care: Reforming Canada's Health System in an Age of Restraint*, Toronto, C. D. Howe Institute, 1994; David Gratzer, *Code Blue: Reviving Canada's Health Care System*, Toronto, ECW Press, 1999.
15 Theresa Boyle, "Health system crash feared," *The Toronto Star*, February 17, 2000.
16 One idea very popular with the Right is the replacement of public financing of medical care by compulsory personal "medical savings accounts." See Gratzer, *op. cit.*
17 "A prescription for medicare, from MP Dr. Keith Martin," *The Ottawa Citizen*, March 11, 2000.
18 On the issue of who should deliver the service, opinion was more evenly split, however. Fifty-one percent of respondents said that "private-sector businesses [should not be allowed] to operate parts of our health-care system," but 47 percent said they should. But how should this be interpreted? What did they understand by "private-sector businesses"? Did they mean *for*-profit or *non*-profit enterprises, or both? Did the 51 percent of respondents mean that there should be less private provision of services, or even none at all? Or did they mean that there should be no *additional* private involvement, beyond the existing private share of financing and service delivery? Similarly, did the 47 percent who said that private-sector businesses should have a role mean that the status quo should prevail, or did they advocate *privatization*, i.e. changing the mixed economy of health care in favour of the private for-profit sector?
19 See Ed Finn (ed.), *The Deficit Made Me Do It*, Ottawa, CCPA, 1993; Ed Finn and Duncan Cameron, *Ten Deficit Myths*, Ottawa, CCPA, 1995.
20 Pat Armstrong, "Privatization," presentation to the Ontario Health Coalition, Toronto, November 1997.
21 The *alternative federal budgets* published by the Canadian Centre for Policy Alternatives and CHO!CES: A Coalition for Social Justice since 1995 have demonstrated this for the federal government. The *alternative Ontario budgets* co-ordinated by the Ontario Federation of Labour have done the same for Ontario.
22 The vigorous resistance of the citizens of Alberta to their government's Bill 11 is a striking example of this.

Chapter 1

1. Michael Rachlis, *A Review of the Alberta Private Hospital Proposal*, Ottawa, Caledon Institute of Social Policy, March 2000, 3. Deber et al. point out in their report to the National Forum on Health: "The literature and international experience both strongly suggest that public or quasi-public single-source financing of health services is optimal, not only on equity grounds, but to achieve cost containment. First, administrative costs are far lower in single-payer systems than in health systems with multiple, competing insurers. Second, there is little incentive to try to shift the cost of care for high-risk, elderly, or other high-cost patients onto other payers. Thus, the inevitable inequities of unequal insurance coverage resulting from multiple insurers are avoided. Third, with one tax-based public insurance system, the costs of financing health care are more evenly distributed throughout the economy—no one particular sector carries the bulk of the financial burden. In countries that rely on employers to pay premiums for their workers, the disincentive of the heavy cost burden for each person added to a payroll is thought to increase unemployment, while people with good medical benefits may be reluctant to change jobs and risk interruption or loss of coverage. Fourth, with one public insurance system, the single payer retains monopsony (single purchaser) bargaining power over service providers, which it can use (should it choose to do so) to achieve greater control over total health care expenditures. This last feature clearly has disadvantages for providers, who will find it more difficult to evade cost controls. (...) In light of these advantages of a single source of financing, most reasons advanced in favour of allowing competing insurers or financers appear to be based on ideology rather than evidence." (*Op. cit.*, 442-443.)
2. Karl Polanyi, *The Great Transformation*, Boston, Beacon Press, 1957.
3. Samuel Martin, *An Essential Grace*, Toronto, McClelland and Stewart, 1985, 27. Having said this, it is of course clear that social citizenship remains an *ideal* that has yet to be fully realized in any country, although some (Sweden being the model usually cited) have come much closer than others.
4. Gøsta Esping-Andersen, "The Three Political Economies of the Welfare State," *Canadian Review of Sociology and Anthropology*, 26:1 (February 1989), 21. See also Gøsta Esping-Andersen, "Citizenship and Socialism: De-Commodification and Solidarity in the Welfare State," in Martin Rein, Gøsta Esping-Andersen, and Lee Rainwater (eds.),

Stagnation and Renewal in Social Policy: The Rise and Fall of Policy Regimes, London, M.E. Sharpe, 1987, 78-101.

5   Esping-Andersen, "The Three Political Economies of the Welfare State."

6   "Scholars have tended to describe post-war welfare states in terms of their impact on the wage relation, categorizing them according to their capacity for 'de-commodifying' labour. Nonetheless, the post-war decades, in which new social policies and new state-society relations were constructed, were also ones in which caring and responsibility for care occupied policy-makers. Providing health care was at the core of post-war welfare state development and competing visions of state-society relations. As Julia O'Connor recently wrote, 'the welfare state is about the care of dependent people. The crisis of the welfare state is at least in part (...) a "crisis of the care of the dependent."'

"In the traditional welfare state literature, however, such programs have been treated as secondary, following *from* the fact that the wage relation was regulated and capital-labour post-war compromises were in place. The profound error of neglecting to see that the 'other' programs were at least as much constitutive of post-war welfare states became evident exactly at the moment that the latter were remodelled in the 1980s and 1990s. There has been an explosion of attention to the 'caring dimensions' of social policies. It has, in other words, become very visible, whereas before it was often hidden in the household or performed in large institutions organized according to the traditional labour processes of Fordism." (Jane Jenson and Susan D. Phillips, "Distinctive Trajectories: Home Care and the Voluntary Sector in Quebec and Ontario," in Keith Banting (ed.)., *The Non-Profit Sector in Canada: Roles and Relationships*, Kingston, Queen's University School of Policy Studies, 2000, 31.)

7   These comments on the three ideologies of health care are inspired by Jan Angus and Ivy Lynn Bourgeault, "Medical Dominance, Gender and the State: The Nurse Practitioner Initiative in Ontario," in David Coburn, Susan Rappolt, Ivy Lynn Bourgeault and Jan Angus, *Medicine, Nursing and the State* [first published as *Health Professions and the State in Ontario*, a special issue of *Health and Canadian Society*, 5:1 (1998-1999)], Toronto, Garamond, 1999, 60.

8   Claus Offe, *Contradictions of the Welfare State*, Cambridge, Mass., MIT Press, 1984. See also James O'Connor, *The Fiscal Crisis of the State*, New York, St. Martin's Press, 1973. On the limits of the Offe/O'Connor analysis as applied to Canada, see Phillip Hansen and Harold Chorney, "The Falling Rate of Legitimation," *Toward a Humanist Political Economy*, Montreal, Black Rose Books, 1992, 72-100.

9   The literature on the crisis of the welfare state is colossal. Recent Canadian contributions include Ramesh Mishra, "After Globalization: Social Policy in an Open Economy," *Canadian Review of Social Policy*, 43 (Spring 1999), 13-28; Margaret Hillyard Little, "The Limits of Canadian Democracy: The Citizenship Rights of Poor Women," *Canadian Review of Social Policy*, 43 (Spring 1999), 59-76; Murray Dobbin, *The Myth of the Good Corporate Citizen: Democracy Under the Rule of Big Business*, Toronto, Stoddart, 1998; Tony Clarke, *Silent Coup: Confronting the Big Business Takeover of Canada*, Ottawa/Toronto, Canadian Centre for Policy Alternatives/Lorimer, 1997; Ken Collier, *After the Welfare State*, Vancouver, New Star Books, 1997; Stephen McBride and John Shields, *Dismantling a Nation: The Transition to Corporate Rule in Canada*, 2nd edition, Halifax, Fernwood Publishing, 1997; Gideon Rosenbluth and Jim Stanford, *The Keynesian Welfare State*, Vancouver, Canadian Centre for Policy Alternatives, 1997; Isabella Bakker (ed.), *Rethinking Restructuring: Gender and Change in Canada*, Toronto, University of Toronto Press, 1996; Robert Boyer and Daniel Drache, *States Against Markets: The Limits of Globalization*, London, Routledge, 1996; Gary Teeple, *Globalization and the Decline of Social Reform*, Toronto, Garamond Press, 1995; Andrew Johnson, Stephen McBride and Patrick J. Smith (eds.), *Continuities and Discontinuities: The Political Economy of Social Welfare and Labour Market Policy in Canada*, Toronto, University of Toronto Press, 1994; Ramesh Mishra, *The Welfare State in Capitalist Society*, Hemel Hempstead, Harvester Wheatsheaf, 1990.

10 See Rodney Haddow, *Poverty Reform in Canada, 1958-1978: State and Class Influences on Policy Making*, Montreal, McGill-Queen's University Press, 1993.

11 See Claus Offe, *op. cit.*

12 This is discussed for example by Leo Panitch and Colin Leys, *The End of Parliamentary Socialism: From New Left to New Labour*, London, Verso, 1997.

13 Ekos Research Associates, "Rethinking Government: Understanding Conflicting Priorities on Tax Cuts, Social Spending and Productivity", Ottawa, August 20, 1999.

14 On the economics of the fiscal crisis, see Jim Stanford, "Over the Rainbow: The Balanced Budget, How We Got It, and How to Hang Onto It," in *Alternative Federal Budget Papers 1998*, Ottawa/Winnipeg, Canadian Centre for Policy Alternatives/CHO!CES, 1998, 325-334; "Economists' Round Table," ibid., 224-275; Jim Stanford, "Disappearing Deficits and Incredible Interest Rates," in *Alternative Federal Budget Papers 1997*, Ottawa/Winnipeg, Canadian Centre for Policy Alternatives/CHO!CES, 1997, 219-274; Jim Stanford, "Growth,

Interest and Debt," ibid., 275-292; Harold Chorney, *The Deficit and Debt Management: Alternatives to Monetarism*, Ottawa, Canadian Centre for Policy Alternatives, 1993. On the politics of deficitism, see Michelle Weinroth, "Deficitism and Neo-Conservatism in Ontario," in Diana Ralph, André Régimbald and Nérée St-Amand (eds.), *Open for Business, Closed to People: Mike Harris's Ontario*, Halifax, Fernwood Publishing, 1997, 54-67; and by the same author, "The Drama of the Deficit," *Canadian Forum*, October 1995, and "Nationalist Ideology in Economic Disguise," *Briarpatch*, September 1994.

[15] Jane Jenson, "'Different' but not 'Exceptional': Canada's Permeable Fordism," *Canadian Review of Sociology and Anthropology*, 26:1 (February 1989), 69-94.

[16] Ibid., 81.

[17] Ibid., 82-83.

[18] On the crisis of federal-provincial relations in the context of the crisis of the welfare state, see for example Paul Leduc Browne (ed.), *Finding Our Collective Voice: Options for a New Social Union*, Ottawa, Canadian Centre for Policy Alternatives, 1998.

[19] Colleen Fuller provides a useful sketch of the origins and development of medicare in her book, *Caring for Profit, op. cit.*

[20] Keith Banting, "Federalism, Social Reform and the Spending Power," *Canadian Public Policy*, XIV, 1988, p. 82.

[21] These are of course the five fundamental principles enshrined in the Canada Health Act, the purpose of which is to "establish criteria and conditions in respect of insured health services and extended health care services provided under provincial law that must be met before a full cash contribution may be made" by the federal government. (Health Canada, *Canada Health Act Annual Report, 1997-1998*, Ottawa, Public Works and Government Services Canada, 1998, 2.)

[22] Originally known as the *Federal-Provincial Fiscal Arrangements and Established Programs Financing Act, 1977*.

[23] The tax room transferred consists of 13.5 personal income tax points and 1.0 corporate income tax points.

[24] National Union of Public and General Employees, "Brief to the Standing Committee on Human Resources Development," March 1994. In its original form, the tax point and cash transfer parts of EPF worked independently of each other. Under a 1982 amendment to the EPF formula "the cash component of the transfer was no longer calculated independently of the tax and equalization components. Under the new formula, the total contribution was calculated, and the population and GNP escalator factors were applied. The cash contribution was then determined as a residual, after subtracting the tax point formula from that total." (*Ibid.*)

25. Ibid.
26. *Funding Health and Higher Education: Danger Looming*, Ottawa, National Council of Welfare, 1991. See also Leslie Seidle, "Financing Health Care and Post-Secondary Education," in Sherri Torjman, *Fiscal Federalism for the 21st Century*, Ottawa, Caledon Institute for Social Policy, 1993, 27-36.
27. *NUPGE News*, "Strange Days: Fiscal Federalism Revisited," 8.
28. *1994 Ontario Budget*, Toronto, Ministry of Finance, 1994, 17. Ontario was worse off than Quebec, because its social assistance benefits were more generous and its social assistance recipients more numerous, but it was receiving only 58 cents from Ottawa for each dollar it spent, while Quebec was getting one dollar. It should however be noted that by virtue of the changes to the Canada Health and Social Transfer announced in the 1999 federal budget, Ontario will in the future be receiving much more per social assistance recipient from Ottawa than Quebec will. This is because Ottawa has moved to equalize the per capita transfer to each province under the CHST. However, the social assistance component of this is no longer pegged to provincial needs, but is in effect a residual amount left over after health care and post-secondary education have been paid for. To be sure, Quebec could choose to pay more for its welfare system and less for health care or post-secondary education. But such a choice is unlikely, given the greater political popularity of the latter programs.
29. CUPE Research Department, *Undoing Health Care: The Canada Health and Social Transfer and How the 1995 Federal Budget Will Affect Medicare*, Ottawa, Canadian Union of Public Employees, 1995.
30. *The Budget Plan*, Ottawa, Department of Finance, 1998; *The Budget Plan*, Ottawa, Department of Finance, 1999; *The Budget Plan*, Ottawa, Department of Finance, 2000.
31. *The 1999 Ontario Alternative Budget*, 2.
32. Parts of this section are borrowed from my "Déjà Vu: Thatcherism in Ontario," in Diana Ralph, André Régimbald and Nérée St-Amand (eds.), *op. cit.*
33. Ian Gough, "Thatcherism and the Welfare State," in Stuart Hall and Martin Jacques (eds.), *The Politics of Thatcherism*, London, Lawrence & Wishart in association with *Marxism Today*, 1983, 154-155.
34. *The Common Sense Revolution*, Toronto, Ontario PC Party, 1994, 1.
35. "Total spending will be reduced by 20 percent in three years, without touching a penny of Health Care funding." (Ibid., 3.)
36. Ibid, passim. See also Ray McLellan, "Alternative Service Delivery in Ontario: The New Public Management," Notes N-11, Toronto, Ontario Legislative Library, Legislative Research Service, January 1997.

37 Ontario, Management Board Secretariat, *Alternative Service Delivery Framework*, Toronto, July 1996, 3. See also Ray McClellan, *op. cit.*, as well as the *Guide to Preparing a Business Case for Alternative Service Delivery* (July 1996), Toronto, Queen's Printer for Ontario, 1997, and Danièle Bélanger, *Alternative Modes of Service Delivery: Information Kit for the Francophone Non-Profit Sector*, Toronto, Office of Francophone Affairs, 1997.

38 "Our vision for the OPS [Ontario Public Service] of the future reflects a strategic refocusing of the core mission of government. The vision is of a public service organization that is:
- focussed on core business;
- ensuring quality service to the public;
- smaller and more flexible;
- integrated and cohesive; and
- accountable.

"Over the past two years, we have come a long way in working towards that vision. Restructuring of the OPS is well under way, and a new framework for government in Ontario is emerging. The framework is one that includes:
- a business planning process in every ministry that links into an overall OPS vision;
- a range of alternative service delivery options that has a focus on the customer, rather than on the provider of service;
- use of the latest technologies to link common service networks and improve access to government;
- major corporate initiatives to re-engineer administrative process across government; and
- performance measures that track how we are doing at the level of the individual, the program, the ministry and the whole organization."

(Rita Burak, *Building the Ontario Public Service for the Future: A Framework for Action*, Toronto, Ontario Public Service Restructuring Secretariat, Cabinet Office, June 1997, quoted in John Shields and B. Mitchell Evans, *Shrinking the State: Globalization and Public Administration "Reform"*, Halifax, Fernwood Publishing, 1998, 115.)

39 Danièle Bélanger, *op. cit.*, 4.
40 Ibid., 5.
41 Ibid., 3-13.
42 See Peter Aucoin, *The New Public Management: Canada in Comparative Perspective*, Montreal, Institute for Research on Public Policy, 1995; Leslie Seidle, *Rethinking the Delivery of Public Services to Citizens*, Montreal, Institute for Research on Public Policy, 1995; David Osborne

and Ted Gaebler, *Reinventing Government: How the Entrepreneurial Spirit Is Transforming the Public Sector*, New York, Penguin Books, 1993.

43 "Does the program area or activity continue to serve a public interest? Is there a legitimate and necessary role for government in this program area or activity? Is the current role of the federal government appropriate, or is the program a candidate for realignment with the provinces? What activities or programs should or could be transferred in whole or in part to the private or voluntary sector? If the program or activity continues, how could its efficiency be improved? Is the resulting package of programs and activities affordable within the fiscal restraint? If not, what programs or activities should be abandoned?" (Quoted by Shields and Evans, *op. cit.*, 48.)

44 Osborne and Gaebler, *op. cit.*, 19-20.

45 Note too that in Ontario "under the New Democratic government, all deputy ministers were issued personal copies of *Reinventing Government*." (Shields and Evans, *op. cit.*, 87.)

46 Paul G. Thomas, "Visions Versus Resources in the Federal Program Review," in Amelita Armit and Jacques Bourgault (eds.), *Hard Choices or No Choices: Assessing Program Review*, Toronto, Institute of Public Administration of Canada, 1996, 46, quoted by Shields and Evans, *op. cit.*, 48.

47 See Shields and Evans, *op. cit.*, 36ff. "The fundamental message of the 'reinventing government' school is that the creation and delivery of public goods must be transformed. The public service must return to focus upon only its core business. In short, the government's core role is to set policy, while the delivery function can best be left to organizations either outside of the state sector or operating under quasi-market conditions within a reorganized public sector. In a general sense, this transformation originated in the collapse of national Keynesian strategies and models and in the political success of neo-liberalism. Consequently, governments are no longer viewed 'as the principal vehicle for socio-economic development' but rather as facilitators of market-led development." (Ibid., 104.)

48 Robin Murray, "Transforming the 'Fordist' State," in Gregory Albo, David Langille and Leo Panitch (eds.), *A Different Kind of State? Popular Power and Democratic Administration*, Toronto, Oxford University Press, 1993, 51-52.

49 George M. Torrance, "Socio-Historical Overview: The Development of the Canadian Health System," in David Coburn, Carl D'Arcy, and George M. Torrance (eds.), *Health and Canadian Society: Sociological Perspectives*, 3rd edition, Toronto, University of Toronto Press, 1998, 5.

50 See George M. Torrance, "Hospitals as Health Factories," in Coburn, D'Arcy and Torrance, *op. cit.*, 438-455; Pat and Hugh Armstrong et al., *Medical Alert*, Toronto, Garamond Press, 1994.

51 On post-fordism, see Alain Lipietz, *Choisir l'audace. Une alternative pour le vingt et unième siècle*, Paris, La Découverte, 1989; David Harvey, *The Condition of Postmodernity*, London, Blackwell, 1989. For thoughts on how this analysis applies to social services, see my article "Post-Social-Democracy, or the Dialectic of the Social Economy," in Dave Broad and Wayne Antony (eds.), *Citizens or Consumers? Social Policy in a Market Society*, Halifax, Fernwood Publishing, 1999, 206-211.

52 Ontario Ministry of Health, *Business Plan*, Toronto, Government of Ontario, May 1996.

53 Having said this, it is important to bear in mind however that in stating that its agenda was to integrate the system, stress prevention and health promotion, substitute community care for hospital care, and so on, the Harris government was not saying anything very different than its Liberal and New Democrat predecessors. As noted above, the Rae government also subscribed to Osborne and Gaebler's vision of "reinventing government."

54 The HSRC's vision document can be found at <http://www.hsrc-crss.org/vision.htm>.

55 Paul Bélanger and Benoît Lévesque, "Le mouvement social au Québec: continuité et rupture (1960-1985)," in Paul R. Bélanger, Benoît Lévesque, Réjean Mathieu and Franklin Midy (eds.), *Animation et culture en mouvement. La fin d'une époque?* Sillery, Presses de l'Université du Québec, 1987, 260ff.; Leo Panitch, "A Different Kind of State?" and Hilary Wainwright, "A New Kind of Knowledge for a New Kind of State," in Albo, Langille and Panitch (eds.), *op. cit.*; Hilary Wainwright, *Arguments for a New Left. Answering the Free-Market Right*, Oxford, Blackwell, 1994.

56 Bélanger and Lévesque, 261.

57 George M. Torrance, "Socio-Historical Overview: The Development of the Canadian Health System," 5.

58 See Robin Murray, *op. cit.*; Guy Roustang et al., *Vers un nouveau contrat social*, Paris, Desclée de Brouwer, 1996; Jean-Louis Laville et al., *Les services de proximité en Europe*, Paris, Syros, 1993; Benoît Lévesque, "Repenser l'économie pour contrer l'exclusion sociale: de l'utopie à la nécessité," in Benoît Lévesque and Juan-Luis Klein (eds.), *Contre l'exclusion. Repenser l'économie*, Sainte-Foy, Presses de l'Université du Québec, 1995, 17-44; Paul Leduc Browne, *Love in a Cold World? The Voluntary Sector in an Age of Cuts*, Ottawa, Canadian Centre for Policy Alternatives, 1996.

59 Ted Allan and Sydney Gordon, *The Scalpel, the Sword*, Toronto, McClelland and Stewart, 1971.

60 Louis Favreau and Benoît Lévesque, *Développement économique communautaire. Économie sociale et intervention*, Sainte-Foy, Presses de l'Université du Québec, 1996; Brian Burtch, *The Trials of Labour: The Re-emergence of Midwifery*, Montreal/Kingston, McGill-Queen's University Press, 1994.

61 Monica Townson, *Health and Wealth: How Social and Economic Factors Affect our Well- Being*, Ottawa/Toronto, Canadian Centre for Policy Alternatives/Lorimer, 1999, 1-2. See also Robert Evans and Gregory Stoddart, "Producing Health, Consuming Health Care," in Coburn, D'Arcy and Torrance, *op. cit.*, 549-579.

62 See for example Richard Wilkinson's *Unhealthy Societies: The Afflictions of Inequality*, London, Routledge, 1996; Robert Chernomas, *The Social and Economic Causes of Disease*, Winnipeg, Canadian Centre for Policy Alternatives, 1999; *Healthy Families: First Things First. The 2000 Alternative Federal Budget*, Ottawa/Winnipeg, Canadian Centre for Policy Alternatives/CHO!CES, 2000; and the Canadian Auto Workers' anti-cancer campaign.

63 "Health is not simply the absence of disease; increasingly, it is being defined as a 'resource for everyday living' (World Health Organization). Indeed, environmental awareness has resulted in linking the health of the individual to the health of the planet. As noted, this expansion of the definition of health has shifted the emphasis from equality of access to medical care to equity of access to health. Given that most policies have health implications, this broad definition presents the health care system with the challenge of determining and defining their boundaries in fulfilling this goal. Health is affected by poverty; does this mean that health policy should shift its attention from hospital and medical services to income distribution, housing, diet, education, environment, and employment? An example of taking such a broad definition can be seen in the *Health for All Ontario—Report of the Panel for Health Goals for Ontario* (Ontario Ministry of Health, 1987). This report concludes that 'society has a collective responsibility to ensure equity through its public policies and its allocation of resources,' and draws from this a powerful agenda for action, stating that 'government action is required to reduce the unacceptable risks to health which are experienced by many Ontarians.' Among the programs advocated are 'affirmative action to enable the disadvantaged to reach their potential'; 'provision of affordable housing, rigorous enforcement of pollution controls, and ensuring of safe workplaces'; elimination of all user fees and reduction of other barriers to access; and empowerment of local commu-

nities and transfer of decision-making authority to the local level." (Sharmila L. Mhatre and Raisa Deber, "From Equal Access to Health Care to Equitable Access to Health: A Review of Canadian Provincial Health Commissions and Reports," in Coburn, D'Arcy and Torrance, *op. cit.*, 465-466.

64 "The insured health services defined by the *Canada Health Act* include all medically necessary hospital services and medically required physician services, as well as medically or dentally required surgical-dental services requiring a hospital for their proper performance. Extended health care services as specified in the *Canada Health Act*, means nursing home intermediate care, adult residential care, home care and ambulatory health care." (Health Canada, *Canada Health Act Annual Report, 1997-1998*, Ottawa, Public Works and Government Services Canada, 1998, 2.)

65 Pat Armstrong, "Privatizing Care," in Pat Armstrong et al, *Medical Alert*, Toronto, Garamond Press, 1997, 15.

66 Ibid., 14.

67 Colleen Fuller, *Caring for Profit: How Corporations Are Taking Over Canada's Health Care System*, Ottawa, Canadian Centre for Policy Alternatives/Vancouver: New Star Books, 1998, 231.

68 See public relations documents produced by the OHA, such as *Partnering for Success: How Health Networks Will Work For You*, or consultants' reports, such as *Health Networks—Seven Case Studies: A Description and Preliminary Analysis*, prepared by KPMG for the OHA. See also *The Hospital-Home Care Interface: Current State and Future Opportunities*, December 1998. All of these documents can be found on the OHA's web site, www.oha.com

69 Robin Murray, "Ownership, Control and the Market," *New Left Review*, 164, July-August 1987.

70 Ibid.

Chapter 2

1 Health economist Raisa Deber of the University of Toronto commenting on the statement by Health Minister Elizabeth Witmer that she had not found any vision of health care in her department on becoming minister. (Art Chamberlain, "In search of a health care road map," *The Toronto Star*, February 22, 1998, F5.)

2 *The Toronto Star*, July 22, 1995.

3 Ontario Ministry of Finance, *Fiscal and Economic Statement*, November 1995.

4 *1996 Ontario Budget: Budget Papers*, Toronto, Ministry of Finance, 1996.

5   *The Common Sense Revolution*, 7.
6   "Health Care Spending on the Rise: CIHI Report," *CIHI Directions*, 6:4 (January 2000).
7   Bill Murnighan, "Health Care Spending in Ontario," Ontario Alternative Budget Working Group, Paper No. 8, April 2000, 6-7.
8   Ibid., 7.
9   *National Health Expenditure Trends, 1975-1998*, Ottawa, Canadian Institute for Health Information, 1998.
10 *Fiscal and Economic Statement*.
11 Ontario Hospital Association, 1999.
12 *The Daily*, Ottawa, Statistics Canada, February 24, 1999.
13 Patricia Tully and Étienne Saint-Pierre, "Downsizing Canada's Hospitals, 1986-1987 to 1994-1995," *Health Reports* (Statistics Canada), 8:4 (Spring 1997), 33. Tully and Saint-Pierre add: "Public sector concern with controlling hospital expenditures is widespread. For this reason, trends in the administration of hospital care are similar in most provinces. The number of approved beds and staffed beds is declining, and hospital stays are becoming shorter. Increasingly, outpatient treatment is favoured, and patients are hospitalized less and less. In addition, operating expenses have levelled off." (Ibid., 39.)
14 In March 2000, the Canadian Institute for Health Information reported that the hospital discharge rate in 1997-1998 was 3 percent lower than in 1996-1997 and 14 percent lower than in 1994-1995. The one-year change was greatest in Ontario—5.3 percent. ("Canada's elderly primary users of hospitals reports Canadian Institute for Health Information," media release, Ottawa, Canadian Institute for Health Information, March 29, 2000.)
15 Ibid.
16 *The Hospital Report '98: A System-wide Review of Ontario's Hospitals*, Toronto, Ontario Hospital Association, 1999, 88.
17 *Fiscal and Economic Statement; 1999 Annual Report Provincial Auditor of Ontario*, 155.
18 Robert K. Muir, "OHA Perspective on the Status of Laboratory Restructuring in Ontario," Toronto, Ontario Hospital Association, January 20, 2000 (this can be found on the OHA web site at <www.oha.com>).
19 Health Services Restructuring Commission, *Final Report on Hospital Restructuring* (this report can be found on the HSRC's web site, <www.hsrc-crss.org>).
20 Kate Bezanson and Louise Noce (with the assistance of the *Speaking Out* Team), *Costs, Closures and Confusion: People in Ontario Talk About*

Health Care, Ottawa, Caledon Institute, *Speaking Out* Project: Periodic Report #4, May 1999, 8.
21. Robert K. Muir, *op. cit.*
22. *1999 Annual Report of the Provincial Auditor of Ontario*, 156.
23. See Dennis Raphael, "Health Effects of Economic Equality: Overview and Purpose," *Canadian Review of Social Policy*, 44 (1999), 25-40; Monica Townson, *Health and Wealth*; Ichiro Kawachi, Bruce P. Kennedy and Richard C. Wilkinson, *The Society and Population Health Reader. Vol. 1: Income Inequality and Health*, New York, The New Press, 1999.
24. Kathryn Wilkins and Evelyn Park, "Characteristics of Hospital Users," *Health Reports* (Statistics Canada), 9:3 (Winter 1997), 35.
25. Gordon Guyatt, "Duncan Sinclair meets with MRG," *Medical Reform* (newsletter of the Medical Reform Group), 17:3 (December 1997), 2.
26. Christel A. Woodward, Harry S. Shannon, Charles Cunningham, John McIntosh, Bonnie Lendrum, David Rosenbloom and Judy Broom, "The Impact of Re-Engineering and Other Cost Reduction Strategies on the Staff of a Large Teaching Hospital," *Medical Care*, 37:6 (1999), 557. On hospital restructuring in general, see Pat Armstrong et al., *Medical Alert*; and Pat and Hugh Armstrong, *Wasting Away: The Undermining of Canadian Health Care*, Toronto, Oxford University Press, 1996.
27. Y. Lilian Chan and Bernadette E. Lynn, "Operating in Turbulent Times: How Ontario's Hospitals Are Meeting the Current Funding Crisis," *Health Care Management Review*, 23:3 (1998), 7.
28. Ibid., 10.
29. *1999 Annual Report of the Provincial Auditor of Ontario*.
30. Ibid.
31. Registered Nurses Association of Ontario/Registered Practical Nurses Association of Ontario, *Ensuring the Care Will Be There: Report on Nursing Recruitment and Retention in Ontario*, Submitted to the Ontario Ministry of Health and Long-Term Care, March 2000, 44.
32. Chan and Lynn, 14. See also *Cooking Up a Storm: Shared Food Services in the Health Care Sector*, Ottawa, CUPE Research Branch, March 1996.
33. Colleen Fuller, *Caring for Profit*, 232.
34. Chan and Lynn, 15.
35. Robert K. Muir, *op. cit.*
36. Med-Chem Health Care Ltd. had previously been the third of the big three laboratory testing company. However, it went bankrupt in 1999 and its assets were acquired in their entirety by Canadian Medical Laboratories Ltd. (CML) in April 1999, making CML the "largest provider of laboratory services in Ontario with a market share of

approximately 33 percent," according to its President and CEO, Dr. John Mull. ("CML Announces Completion of Acquisition of Substantially All of the Laboratory Assets of Med-Chem Health Care Limited," *Canada News Wire*, April 16, 1999; "The Ontario Association of Medical Laboratories Announces Further Increase in Funding for Laboratory Services," *Canada News Wire*, May 14, 1999.)

37 *Medical Lab Services: Public vs. Private Delivery Systems*, Nepean, National Union of Public and General Employees, revised edition, May 1997, 5. This document points out that "private laboratory owners have moved aggressively toward low-unit-cost/high-volume testing involving the development of large automated centralized testing facilities. To support efficiency and profitability of their operation, each centralized testing facility is linked to a large specimen collection network in order to provide the required volume of test requests. Full advantage is taken of communications technology to return test results to requesting clinicians and to keep turnaround time within acceptable limits." (Ibid.)

38 Ibid., 2.
39 Ibid., 6.
40 Ibid., 10.
41 Ibid., 9.
42 Jonathan Forbes, *Test Case: Private vs. Public Laboratories*, North York, Ontario Public Service Employees Union, 1996, 4. A schedule was established under Regulation 552 of the *Health Insurance Act* to enable OHIP to claw back the excess payments.
43 "The Ontario Association of Medical Laboratories Announces Further Increase in Funding for Laboratory Services," *Canada News Wire*, May 14, 1999.
44 Terence Corcoran, "Ontario Tories fail lab test," *The Globe and Mail*, May 27, 1998.
45 Ibid.
46 Jonathan Forbes, *op.cit.*, passim.
47 Ibid.
48 Canadian Union of Public Employees, *When Seniors Don't Matter*, Toronto, 1999.
49 RNAO/RPNAO, *Ensuring the Care Will Be There*, 61, 62, 65.
50 Canadian Union of Public Employees, *When Seniors Don't Matter*, Toronto, 1999.
51 J. Shannan and B. Chatmers, *Nurse Effectiveness: Health and Cost-Effectiveness of Nursing Services*, Report of the World Health Organization Collaborating Centre for International Nursing Development in Leadership Administration and Clinical Practice, 1996, 11 (cited

in the joint statement of the Registered Nurses Association and Ontario Nurses Association, *Replacement of Registered Nurses by Less Prepared Providers*, December 1996).
52 M. Bryant, A. Frost, B. Golden, K. Hardy and P. Newson, *Leading the Management of Change: A Study of Twelve Ontario Hospitals*, Ivey School of Business, University of Western Ontario, report released by the OHA, 1997, cited by Woodward et al., 557.
53 Ibid, 564.
54 RNAO/RPNAO, *Ensuring the Care Will Be There*, 54.
55 *Good Nursing, Good Health: An Investment in the 21st Century*, Report of the Nursing Task Force, Toronto, Ministry of Health of Ontario, 1999.
56 Ibid.
57 "Nursing for Hospitals," *Canada News Wire*, March 19, 1999 (Ontario Ministry of Health, press release). "Backgrounder—Ministry of Health Response to Nursing Task Force," Toronto, Ontario Ministry of Health, March 1999.
58 "Backgrounder—Ministry of Health Response to Nursing Task Force," Toronto, Ontario Ministry of Health, March 1999.
59 *The Toronto Star*, March 19, 1999, A18.
60 *The Toronto Star*, March 25, 1999.
61 *Canadian Press*, August 5, 1999.
62 RNAO/RPNAO, *Ensuring the Care Will Be There*.
63 *The Toronto Star*, December 8, 1998, A16.
64 Institutions to which the government extended the status of Crown Foundation included the Ontario Cancer Treatment and Research Foundation, the Ontario Arts Council, the Art Gallery of Ontario, the Royal Ontario Museum, the Royal Botanical Garden, the National Ballet of Canada, the Canadian Opera Company, the Toronto Symphony Orchestra, the Shaw Festival, the Stratford Festival, public hospitals, and public libraries.
65 "A Crown foundation is nothing more than a legal mechanism for processing large donations relative to a person's income." (Ontario, Legislative Assembly, Hansard: Official Report of Debates, 36th Parliament, 1st Session [19 June 1996], 3776, quoted by David Rampersad, "Alternative Sources of Funding for Public Institutions in Ontario," Backgrounder 28, Toronto, Ontario Legislative Library, January 1999.)
66 Ibid.
67 Ibid.
68 Paul Leduc Browne, *Love in a Cold World?* 53ff.
69 "With the prevalence of the 'free market' ideology today, some people see charity as an improvement over government social spend-

ing. The latter depends on taxes, which are regarded as coercive, while charity is a matter of the donor's voluntary choice. In fact, charity in Canada is not an alternative to government spending. As soon as governments give people tax credits and deductions for making charitable donations, charity involves another form of government spending—a 'tax expenditure.'" (Ibid., 55.)

70 "Health care or culture? Education or social services? Food banks or the Anglican Church? It is a nasty way of posing the alternatives, and Canadian citizens should not be faced with it. Governments should maintain and improve the essential services entrusted to them by the voters by ensuring a sufficient flow of tax revenue and spending the funds on efficient, accountable, professionally run, not-for-profit public services accessible to all. Furthermore, those who provide such services in the voluntary sector should not be wasting time and money trying to raise funds privately to keep their agencies afloat, instead of seeing to their real mission." (Ibid., 56.)

71 "Fact Sheet on Long-Term Care," Ontario Health Coalition web site at <www.web.net/ohc>.

72 Information obtained from the Ontario Ministry of Health web site at <www.gov.on.ca>.

73 Office of the Provincial Auditor of Ontario, *1995 Annual Report*.

74 *The Toronto Star*, March 28, 1996, A1; *The Ottawa Citizen*, March 29, 1996, D11.

75 RNAO/RPNAO, *Ensuring the Care Will Be There*, 41.

76 *The Ottawa Citizen*, May 27, 1998.

77 RNAO/RPNAO, *Ensuring the Care Will Be There*, 42.

78 The 1995 Provincial Auditor's report declared "We found no evidence of any analysis performed by the Ministry to establish the need for this guarantee or to determine the appropriateness of the 2.25-hour minimum standard." It recommended: "Rather than guaranteeing a minimum number of hours, the Ministry should fund nursing and personal care based on an evaluation of care needs." The Ministry responded: "The recommendation to fund based on assessed needs is supported. The results of the resident classification confirm that the provision of 2.25 hours of nursing care does not meet actual resident needs in every facility, and will therefore be reviewed. (Office of the Provincial Auditor of Ontario, *1995 Annual Report*.)

79 Pat Armstrong and Hugh Armstrong, *Women, Privatization and Health Reform: The Ontario Case*, 1999, 29.

80 Registered Nurses' Association of Ontario, 1999.

81 *The Ottawa Citizen*, July 24, 1996, C3.

82 *The Globe and Mail*, March 13, 1997; *The Toronto Star*, March 13, 1997; *The Toronto Sun*, March 13, 1997; *The Toronto Star*, March 14, 1997.
83 *The Globe and Mail*, August 13, 1997.
84 *The Toronto Star*, March 10, 1999, A4.
85 Statement of Health Minister Elizabeth Witmer in the Ontario Legislature, *Debates of the Legislative Assembly of Ontario* (Hansard), April 29, 1998.
86 *The Globe and Mail*, April 30, 1998.
87 Opposition response to the statement by the Minister of Health by Marion Boyd, M.P.P., *Debates of the Legislative Assembly of Ontario (Hansard)*, April 29, 1998.
88 Pat Armstrong and Hugh Armstrong, *Women, Privatization and Health Reform*, 27.
89 *The Globe and Mail*, May 26, 1998.
90 *The Ottawa Citizen*, March 25, 1999.
91 *The Toronto Star*, April 30, 1998.
92 *Ottawa Sun*, October 30, 1998, 8.
93 *The Toronto Star*, November 29, 1998.
94 *Land Ambulance Issues for Ontario's Hospitals*, Ontario Hospital Association, December 1999, 8.
95 Ibid.
96 Ibid.
97 "Ambulance for the past 30 years: public, non-profit," *Privatization Issues*, Ontario Public Service Employees Union (OPSEU) web site, <http://www.opseu.org/privatization/issues.htm>
98 With some exceptions. See Regulation 552 of the *Health Insurance Act*, in *Revised Statutes of Ontario, 1990*.
99 Regulation 552 of the *Health Insurance Act*.
100 "Ambulance Fees," *Emergency Health Services*, Ministry of Health, June 22, 1998.
101 Ministry of Health and Long-Term Care, *"Who Does What" Initiative: Land Ambulance Services*, Government of Ontario web site <http://www.gov.on/health/english/pub/legis/wdwam.html>, December 1997.
102 Summary Notes, Meeting No. 2, Land Ambulance Implementation Steering Committee, March 1999, quoted in *Land Ambulance Issues for Ontario's Hospitals*, 23.
103 "Ambulance for the past 30 years: public, non-profit"; "Bill 152," Brief by the Canadian Union of Public Employees, <http://www.cupe.on.ca/briefs/bill152.html>
104 "Status of Ambulance Downloading to the Municipalities," *Privatization Issues*, Ontario Public Service Employees Union (OPSEU) web site, <http://www.opseu.org/privatization/municipal.htm>

105 OPSEU sources report that Bruce County voted on April 13, 2000, to keep the ambulance service in house, while the City of Cornwall voted on April 25, 2000, to keep the Stormont, Dundas & Glengarry ambulance service in house.
106 *The Globe and Mail*, November 8, 1995, A2; *The Toronto Star*, October 12, 1995, A3.
107 *The Toronto Star*, August 26, 1995.
108 *The Ottawa Citizen*, November 25, 1995, A1; *The Globe and Mail*, November 8, 1995, A1.
109 Data provided by the Ministry of Health and Long-Term Care, April 2000 and drawn from the Public Accounts of Ontario, 1997-1998, 1998-1999.
110 Robert Evans, "Health Reform: What 'Business' Is It of Business?" in Daniel Drache and Terry Sullivan, *op. cit.*, 28.
111 *The Toronto Star*, 12/XII/95, A3.
112 *The Toronto Star*, November 23, 1996, A1.
113 Ministry of Health and Long-Term Care fact sheet, *Chronic Care Co-payment*, 2000 at www.gov.on.ca/MOH/english/pub/chronic/chronic.html. For the calendar of increases, see Regulation 552 of the *Health Insurance Act*.
114 Monica Townson, *A Report Card on Women and Poverty*, Ottawa, Canadian Centre for Policy Alternatives, April 2000, 1.
115 "OHIP Coverage Updated," Ministry of Health and Long-Term Care, News Release, February 24, 1998.
116 The fourteen outmoded procedures removed were:
- "Posturography, a test to assess the patient's sense of balance using a computerized platform;
- "Stapes mobilization, a procedure to improve movement of bones in the ear;
- "Eustachian tube catherization to treat a drainage problem in the inner ear;
- "Typanotomy, a surgical procedure to relieve pressure on the eardrum;
- "Caloric testing (use of hot and cold water on the eardrum) without ENG to diagnose neurological problems;
- "Vidian neurectomy, surgical cutting of a nose nerve to prevent stuffiness not caused by an infection;
- "Oxytocin challenge test, a method of observing fetal heart rates;
- "Automatic tympanometry to measure flexibility of the eardrum;
- "Opening of the dura, the outermost membrane covering the brain and spinal cord;
- "Hypothermia, induced reduction of body temperature for some types of surgery;

- Open reduction-spinal, the correction of a spinal fracture or dislocation after incision to the spine;
- "Cerebral ventriculogram, a technique to show head movement on a single x-ray film;
- "Diagnostic burr-holes, the drilling of a small hole in the skull for diagnostic purposes;
- "Intralesional injections, the injection of synthetic hormones to treat acne."

("Revisions to the OHIP Schedule of Benefits," Ministry of Health and Long-Term Care, February 24, 1998.)

[117] "Revisions to OHIP Schedule of Benefits: Why Has OHIP Coverage Been Reviewed?" Ministry of Health and Long-Term Care Backgrounder, February 24, 1998.

[118] "Fact Sheet: Eye Examination," *OHIP Bulletin, 8076—Fact Sheet*, 1998.

[119] Ontario Health Insurance Plan, *Bulletin*, 4314 (June 30, 1998), 4330 (December 24, 1998).

[120] David Coburn, "Professional Autonomy and the Problematic Nature of Self-Regulation," in David Coburn et al., *Medicine, Nursing and the State*, 27. As Coburn puts it: "the general trend in health care is clear: to rescue government health insurance from its fiscal pressures, medical care is to be rationalized. Furthermore, governments facilitated the rise of a number of different health care disciplines, from economics to epidemiology, whose raison d'être is more science in health care and whose knowledge base is drawn, not necessarily only from a medical science controlled by the medical profession, but from epidemiology, economics, or health administration. Physicians and medical organizations can no longer claim to have exclusive expertise over health care, though still clinging to an increasingly challenged claim to exclusive knowledge over the content of care." (Ibid., 37-38.)

[121] "In the case of physicians, the gatekeepers to medical care, the state first became interested in fee negotiations in an attempt to control costs. When it was discovered that fees could not control costs (partly because the ever-increasing number of physicians could adjust the number and type of procedures given to hit a target income), state policy moved in sequence to cap the incomes of individual physicians at some (large) amount, to reduce physician numbers, and, presently, to both restrict the numbers of physicians and place a cap on the *total* amount which all physicians in the province can bill the government plan (taking into account increases in population, etc.)." (Ibid., 29.)

[122] Ivy Lynn Bourgeault and Jan Argus, "Pay and Human Resource Management in Nursing and Medicine: An Examination of Gendered

Structural Relations Between the Professions and the State," in David Coburn et al., *Medicine, Nursing and the State*, 100.
123 David Coburn, "Professional Autonomy and the Problematic Nature of Self-Regulation," 38.
124 *The Toronto Star*, December 17, 1996; *The Toronto Star*, May 28, 1997.
125 For example, they can order ultrasounds, x-rays and lab tests without the approval of a physician.
126 "Cost-savings result because: 1) practices that employ nurse-practitioners could provide more services for a fixed amount of health care dollars; 2) length of hospital stay could be reduced by having nurse practitioners provide more community care; and 3) it is cheaper to train a nurse-practitioner than it is to train a physician. The level of remuneration for a nurse practitioner is also significantly lower than for a physician." (Jan Argus and Ivy Lynn Bourgeault, "Medical Dominance, Gender and the State: The Nurse Practitioner Initiative in Ontario," 63.
127 Ibid.
128 Ibid.
129 Ibid., 73.
130 *London Free Press*, October 1, 1996, A1.
131 "Ontario Docs Excel at Creative Extra-Billing," *Medical Reform* (Newsletter of the Medical Reform Group), 18:2 (September 1998), 1-2.
132 *The Toronto Star*, June 13, 1995.
133 *The Toronto Star*, April 4, 1998.
134 Gina Feldberg and Robert Vipond, "The Virus of Consumerism," in Daniel Drache and Terry Sullivan (eds.), *op. cit.*, 48-64.
135 *The Globe and Mail*, June 25, 1996; *The Toronto Star*, July 18, 1996; *The Ottawa Citizen*, July 19, 1996; *The Toronto Star*, July 19, 1996; *The Globe and Mail*, July 19, 1996.
136 See for example the vision statement of the Health Services Restructuring Commission cited in Chapter 1. The HSRC also later produced its own detailed road map of how to create such a system, *Primary Health Care Strategy: Advice and Recommendations to the Honourable Elizabeth Witmer, Minister of Health*, December 1999. See the response to it drafted by the Association of Ontario Health Centres, January 2000. See also The College of Family Physicians of Canada, *Managing Change: The Family Medicine Group Practice Model*, September 1995, and *Family Medicine in the 21st Century—A Prescription for Excellence in Health Care*, June 1999; Ontario Medical Association, *Primary Care Reform—A Strategy for Stability*; and Association of Ontario Health Centres, *Community Health Centres: A Cost-Effective Solution to Primary Health Care Reform*, April 2000.
137 *The Ottawa Citizen*, May 26, 1998.

138 *The Ottawa Citizen*, March 5, 1998.
139 Pat and Hugh Armstrong, *Women, Privatization and Health Reform: The Ontario Case*, 35.
140 Ontario Health Coalition, *Newsletter*, May 2000, 1.

Chapter 3

1. Norman Johnson (ed.), *Private Markets in Health and Welfare: An International Perspective*, Oxford, Berg, 1995,10.
2. Quoted by M. Anderson & K. Parent, *Putting a Face on Home Care. CARP's Report on Home Care in Canada 1999*, Kingston, Queen's Health Policy Research Unit, 1999, 8.
3. Ministry of Health, *Health Care Programs. Long-Term Care Community Services*, backgrounder prepared by the Ministry of Health—East Region, update June 1999.
4. *Statutes of Ontario, 1994*, Chapter 26 (*Long-Term Care Act, 1994*), s. 2 (3-7).
5. Peter Coyte and Wendy Young, *Reinvestment in and Use of Home Care Services*, Toronto, Institute for Clinical Evaluative Sciences, November 1997, 3 (emphasis added). Dr. Peter Coyte of the University of Toronto and the Institute for Clinical Evaluative Sciences is co-director of the Home Care Evaluation and Research Centre established at the University of Toronto in 1999.
6. *The Toronto Star*, March 16, 1996, A4.
7. Coyte & Young, *op. cit.*, 3. In an interesting initiative in this context, the Haldimand-Norfolk Community Care Access Centre has established a Nurse Outpatient Clinic at the Norfolk General Hospital. Younger and more mobile patients are encouraged to visit the clinics for dressing changes, catheter care, intravenous therapy or injections, rather than be visited at home by a nurse. Patients are taught at the clinic how to perform some of the care themselves. The hospital bills the Community Care Access Centre (CCAC). According to the CCAC's manager responsible for the project, "a visit to the clinic costs about $10 less than a home care nurse visiting a patient's home." Similar clinics exist in other parts of Ontario. ("Outpatient Service Eases Need for Home Care Workers," *Simcoe Reformer*, reproduced on the web site of the Haldimand-Norfolk Community Care Access Centre, at <http://www.hnccac.on.ca/ccacnews.html>.)
8. "Hospital patients home sooner, cheaper with home care," *A Closer Look*, Health Services Utilization and Research Commission (HSURC), 1998 (summary of the HSURC's *Hospital and Home Care*

Study at <http://www.sdh.sk.ca/hsurc/nlspring98.htm>). Similarly, a recent study by researchers at the University of Leicester in Britain reportedly concludes that home care is not only cheaper than hospital care, but that patients treated at home need only half as many days of care as those treated in hospital. (André Picard, "British report cites advantages of home care," *The Globe and Mail*, December 20, 1999.)

9. The National Evaluation of the Cost-Effectiveness of Home Care, *Newsletter*, 1:1 (2000), at <http://www.homecarestudy.com/newsletter/page1.html>
10. Ibid. (emphasis added).
11. Ibid.
12. Ibid. (emphasis added).
13. Ibid.
14. Ontario Community Support Association, *Pre-Budget Consultation Submission to the Ontario Ministry of Finance*, April 1, 1999.
15. Ontario Home Health Care Providers' Association, *Recruitment and Retention of the Home Care Sector Workforce*, October 1999.
16. Margaret MacAdam, *Human Resource Issues in Home Care in Canada: A Policy Perspective*, Home Care Development, Health Canada, Ottawa, Public Works and Government Services Canada, July 1999.
17. Ontario Community Support Association, *Pre-Budget Submission to the Ontario Ministry of Finance*, April 1, 1999.
18. Conference Board of Canada News Release, "Eldercare taking its toll on Canadian workers," November 10th, 1999; Elizabeth Church, "Number of workers who care for elderly and children rising: study," *The Globe and Mail*, November 11th, 1999, B12. An excellent overview of the question can be found in Pat Armstrong and Hugh Armstrong, *Wasting Away: The Undermining of Canadian Health Care*, 137ff.
19. We Care Health Services, *Survey of Offices*, November 1999.
20. For the distinction between "insured services" and "extended health services," see the *Canada Health Act Annual Report*, Ottawa, Health Canada, 2000.
21. Toronto Community Care Access Centre, *Challenge 2000*, Annual Report, April 1, 1998- March 31, 1999, 7.
22. *Long-Term Care Act, 1994*, Ontario Regulation 386/99, "Provision of Community Services."
23. "Caregiver" is defined in the regulation as "a family member, friend or other person who (a) has primary responsibility for the care of an applicant for homemaking or personal support services or of a per-

24 Ibid.
25 Personal communication from Sharon Marsden of the Ministry of Health and Long-Term Care, April 10, 2000.
26 Kingston, Frontenac, Lennox & Addington Community Care Access Centre, 1999.
27 *Service Directions for CCACs and Other LTC Community Agencies*, draft, Ministry of Health, Long-Term Care Division, January 1999.
28 Health Canada, *Public Home Care Expenditures in Canada, 1975-76 to 1997-98*, at <http://www.hc-sc.gc.ca>; *Expenditure Estimates, 1999-2000*, Toronto, Ministry of Finance, 2000.
29 Interview with the author, April 2000.
30 And provided, to the extent that they had not divested the services.
31 CCPA August-September 1999 survey of CCACs. In surveying the CCACs, we made a commitment not to publish any of the information they provided us in such a way as to make it possible for them to be identified. When I have specifically named them, it is only on the basis of published reports.
32 Heather Kok-Wright, "CCAC watching its bottom-line," *Chatham Daily News*, December 21, 1999.
33 Toronto Community Care Access Centre, *op. cit.*, p. 1.
34 Interview with CCAC case manager, July 1999.
35 Heather Kok-Wright, *op. cit.*
36 Bryan Parker, "Seniors want community care services restored," *Cornwall Standard- Freeholder*, March 2, 2000.
37 "Home Care Agency Calls for Greater Self-Reliance," *Simcoe Reformer*, reproduced on the Haldimand-Norfolk CCAC web site at <http://www.hnccac.on.ca/ccacnews.html>
38 Registered Nurses' Association of Ontario, *Reclaiming a Vision: Making Long-Term Care Community Services Work*, Toronto, September 1999, 6.
39 Pat and Hugh Armstrong, *Wasting Away*; Pat Armstrong, Hugh Armstrong, Jacqueline Choinière, Eric Mykhalovskiy and Jerry P. White, *Medical Alert*.
40 Chris Thompson and Anne Jarvis, "Blind man's dinner sets off alarms," *The Windsor Star*, February 3, 2000.
41 Roseann Danese, "City inherits CCAC clients," *The Windsor Star*, February 7, 2000; Anne Jarvis, "CCAC to seek more funding," *The Windsor Star*, February 28, 2000.
42 Thompson and Jarvis, "Blind man's dinner sets off alarms."

43 Roseann Danese, "City inherits CCAC clients."
44 Myra Conway, "Overview of the Federal Government's Involvement in Home Care: Past and Present," Opening plenary presentation, 8th National Canadian Home Care Association Conference, December 1998. Myra Conway was at the time of the presentation Director of Policy, Home Care Development Unit, Health Canada.
45 Jiajian Chen and Russell Wilkins, "Seniors' Needs for Health-Related Personal Assistance," *Health Reports*, 10:1 (Summer 1998), 49.
46 Ibid., 45.
47 Jane Jenson and Susan D. Phillips, "Distinctive Trajectories," 46, 62.
48 Ibid.
49 *Partnerships in Long-Term Care: A New Way to Plan, Manage, and Deliver Services and Community Support. A Policy Framework*, Ontario, Ministry of Health, April 1993.
50 Minister for Senior Citizens' Affairs, *A New Agenda: Health and Social Service Strategies for Ontario's Seniors*, Government of Ontario, 1989, quoted in Jenson and Phillips, 48.
51 Jenson and Phillips, 48; Howard Litwin and Ernie Lightman, "The Development of Community Care Policy for the Elderly: A Comparative Perspective," *International Journal of Health Services*, 26:4 (1996), 696.
52 *Partnerships in Long-Term Care: A New Way to Plan, Manage, and Deliver Services and Community Support. A Policy Framework*, 24-27.
53 *Partnerships in Long-Term Care: A New Way to Plan, Manage, and Deliver Services and Community Support. An Implementation Framework*, Ontario, Ministry of Health, June 1993, 14. The following qualification was added: "Service agencies that become part of an MSA should not feel that they will be asked to give up their individual identities. It is expected that some agencies, such as those providing ethnocultural services, will retain their identities and unique service aspects." (Ibid., 15.)
54 *The Ottawa Citizen*, March 27, 1997.
55 The parallels between Ontario and other countries are striking: "During the 1980s, the welfare state in the UK and other advanced capitalist states underwent profound changes, driven by both expenditure crises and ideological critiques. The political paradigm of the New Right became dominant, entailing a radical review of the scale and scope of state intervention, especially in social policy. In the UK, as elsewhere, public spending on health care was a cause of major concern, as demand increased, demographic trends intensified claims on resources, and innovations in medical technology extended the

range of possible treatments. Throughout Europe and North America, health-care systems became the target of cost-containment programs and organizational reform.

"The resulting strategy, adopted by many different countries, comprised the application, or restoration, of market principles to formerly publicly financed and publicly provided health-care systems. In the UK, because of widespread political support for the National Health Service (NHS), the Government recognized that outright privatization was not feasible, and so from 1991 introduced a massive restructuring process based on the idea of an 'internal market.' Within a universal, tax-funded system, the provision of health services was separated from purchasing, and competition between hospitals and other provider units was expected to stimulate greater cost-efficiency and improved quality. For this quasi-market to work, it was necessary to implement a complex contracting process to enable purchasers to specify needs and objectives and to negotiate and monitor services, prices and quality with various providers." (Rob Flynn, Gareth Williams, Susan Pickard, *Markets and Networks: Contracting in Community Health Services*, Buckingham, Open University Press, 1996, 1.)

56 August/September 1999 CCPA Survey of CCACs. Jane Jenson and Susan Phillips ("Distinctive Trajectories") suggest that the charitable status of the CCACs is intended to enable them to supplement provincial funding with donations. However, as of the autumn of 1999, they still had not engaged in fund-raising (although some planned to do so) and still received virtually 100 percent of their revenues from the provincial government.

57 August/September 1999 CCPA Survey of CCACs.

58 Letter to the author from the Ministry of Health and Long-Term Care, November 15, 1999.

59 Author's interviews with key informants from the for-profit and non-profit sectors.

60 Margaret MacAdam, *Human Resource Issues in Home Care in Canada: A Policy Perspective.*

61 For a more detailed profile of Olsten, see *The Cost of Privatization: Olsten Corporation and the Crisis in American For-Profit Home Care*, Winnipeg, Canadian Centre for Policy Alternatives—Manitoba, 1997.

62 See the web site of Gentiva Health Services at <www.gentiva.com>.

63 Ontario Home Health Care Providers' Association, *The Competitive Process in Contracting for Home Health and Social Care Provision*, position paper, March 1999, 7.

64 Registered Nurses' Association of Ontario, *Reclaiming a Vision*, 9. The Ontario Home Health Care Providers' Association, representing the for-profit providers, has also voiced a number of criticisms of the RFP process and recommendations for improvement. These are contained in its position paper, *The Competitive Process in Contracting for Home Health and Social Care Provision*.

65 Interview with the author, September 1999.

66 "Provincial Requirements for the Request for Proposal Process for the Provision of In-Home Services, Supplies and Equipment," Toronto, Ministry of Health, Long-Term Care Division, May 1996, 1.

67 I am grateful to Hugh Armstrong for sharing this information with me.

68 Hamilton-Wentworth CCAC web site at <http://www.hwccac/images/RFP%20Schedule.htm>

69 Information gathered at the web site of the Ontario Association of Community Care Access Centres at <http://www.oaccac.on.ca/request.html> in March 2000.

70 *Kitchener-Waterloo Record*, July 24, 1998, A20.

71 Flynn et al, 18.

72 Ibid.

73 *Reclaiming a Vision*, 12.

74 Interview with the author, October 1999.

75 *The Competitive Process in Contracting*, 9.

76 Interview with the author, April 2000.

77 See Shirlee Sharkey and Lesley Larsen, "Supersmart Homes: A New Meaning for Home Care," *Caring Magazine*, October 1999, 26-27; Shirlee Sharkey and Lesley Larsen, "Healthcare Revolution: Led by consumers, fuelled by technology," *Canadian Healthcare Manager*, December 1999/January 2000, 25-27; Shirlee Sharkey, "Following a new leader: Emerging consumerism reshapes community care," *Rehab & Community Care Management*, Spring 2000, 42-43.

78 Flynn et al., 142-143.

79 Ibid., 136.

80 Ibid., 142-143.

81 Ibid., 137.

82 Interview with the author, October 1999.

83 Interview with the author, April 2000.

84 Flynn et al., 139.

85 Ibid., 141.

86 Ibid., 140.

87 Interview with the author, October 1999.

88 Interview with the author, October 1999.
89 Evelyn Shapiro, *The Cost of Privatization: A Case Study of Home Care in Manitoba*, Winnipeg, Canadian Centre for Policy Alternatives, 1997, 5.
90 See Lester B. Salamon, "Partners in Public Service: The Scope and Theory of Government-Nonprofit Relations," in Walter W. Powell (ed.), *The Nonprofit Sector. A Research Handbook*, New Haven, Yale University Press, 1987; Jean-Louis Laville et al., *Les services de proximité en Europe*, Paris, Syros, 1993; Yves Vaillancourt (with Christian Jetté), *Vers un nouveau partage des responsabilités dans les services sociaux et de santé: rôles de l'État, du marché, de l'économie sociale et du secteur informel*, Montreal, Laboratoire de recherche sur les pratiques et les politiques sociales, Université du Québec à Montréal, 1997.
91 Josephine Rekart, *Public Funds, Private Provision: The Role of the Voluntary Sector*, Vancouver, UBC Press, 1993, 22.
92 Ibid., 21.
93 Salamon, 109. Estelle James and Susan Rose-Ackerman explain the concept of "contract failure" thus: "In Hansmann's model, the producer has more information about product quality than the consumer does. Since consumers cannot observe certain quality characteristics, they are unable to monitor them and producers will always have an incentive to cheat. Hence, contracts for these characteristics will not be written or enforced and they will be underproduced and underconsumed in ordinary profit-maximizing markets. The non-distribution constraint allegedly reduces the incentive for the firm to downgrade quality and reassures the consumer that high quality will be maintained. The consumer, finding the non-profit firm more 'trustworthy,' is willing to contract with it for goods whose quality cannot be monitored. NPOs have a comparative advantage in the provision of such goods, and enhance the overall efficiency of the marketplace by enabling them to be produced and consumed." (Estelle James and Susan Rose-Ackerman, *The Non-Profit Enterprise in Market Economics*, New York, Harwood Academic Publishers, 1986, 21.)
94 This is not to claim that the individuals who work in such settings are unscrupulous or unprofessional. It is merely to say that the values of altruism, solidarity, co-operation and service associated with care are contradicted by the basic law governing profit-maximizing corporations.
95 "Health care organizations that are motivated strictly or primarily for-profit behave differently from those with more diverse objectives.

They adopt whatever behaviours will maximize the margins of revenue over cost. A fundamental 'tension between profit maximization and medical appropriateness' is reflected in distortions in patterns of patient management and medical decision-making so as to generate higher margins. In less competitive environments, charges and use of services (whether or not appropriate) tend to be higher among for-profit firms. In more competitive environments, for-profit organizations appear to find ways to reduce their costs of operation and protect their larger operating margins." (Evans et al., *Private Highway, One-Way Street*, 2.)

96 *The Ottawa Citizen*, June 1, 1998, A6.
97 I am not trying to argue simplistically that each and every profit-maximizing business is bad and every non-profit organization is good. Common sense and experience tell us that individuals do not lose all sense of altruism, solidarity or professionalism when they go to work in a profit-maximizing enterprise. It is clear, too, that some not-for-profit agencies are incompetent and corrupt, just as some for-profit businesses provide services of the highest calibre. My point is rather that, in the final analysis, the shareholders of a corporation will require that investment and management decisions be based on profitability above all. There are therefore built-in limits to the range and quality of service such a corporation can provide in the human-services field. Different limits apply to non-profits.
98 Interview with the author, October 1999.
99 *The Toronto Star*, August 26, 1999.
100 Brian Cross, "Successor rights fight set," *The Windsor Star*, May 15, 2000, A4.
101 "Of the 240 nurses who lost their jobs, most have gone on to Windsor or Detroit hospitals or nursing homes. Meanwhile, there's a dire shortage of 130 home-care nurses at the three agencies, basically because they've only been able to attract about 40 of the former VON nurses." (Ibid.)
102 "Staff at Victorian Order of Nurses Simcoe Branch vote to accept insolvency proposal," Press Release, Victorian Order of Nurses Simcoe County Branch, October 13, 1999.
103 Kellie Hudson, "Home care plans hit by cash squeeze," *The Toronto Star*, March 30, 1999
104 According to the former director of VON-Ontario, Herb Pirk: "This notion that everyone is put on an equal playing field is just bullshit. For the VON, for the not-for-profits, it's not managed competition, it's managed decline." (Ibid.)

105 We can speculate as to why the response rate was so much lower for that question than for the others. Possible reasons could include technical or political considerations.

On the technical side, CCACs tally the total number of visits or hours of service provided for their own planning purposes, as well as for the Ministry of Health. It is also fairly simple to compile a list of service providers under contract. However, many CCACs will not have any reason to differentiate between non-profits and for-profits in keeping records of the services they purchase. Our question required them not only to copy out available information, but in many cases no doubt to calculate the figures for the first time. This is a time-consuming task. It is to be expected that the response rate will be much lower when the respondents, who are all very busy and for whom a survey represents an additional and unexpected chore, have to spend much more time answering the questions.

Managed competition is also a politically contentious issue. Some CCACs may have preferred to avoid a question which asked them to differentiate between or compare non-profit and for-profit agencies.

106 See Jenson and Phillips, *op. cit.*, 63-64.

107 Pay equity contains some grey areas. It appears that some for-profit companies may also be covered by it, namely those which were already active in home care when pay equity legislation was passed, while others are not bound by it.

108 *The Globe and Mail*, June 5, 1999, A6.

109 Evelyn Shapiro raised similar concerns in Manitoba: "Why did Olsten Health Services [in Manitoba] agree to a contract which all other eligible companies rejected? Could it be that a large multinational company has the financial resources to afford a 'loss leader' in order to gain a foothold in what might be a lucrative business when other competitors are shut out and prices can then be raised? Such tendering practices are not unknown in the United States where the goal of such companies is to reduce or actually wipe out potential competitors before raising prices." (Evelyn Shapiro, *op.cit.*, 13-14.)

110 This argument was put to the author by the director of a branch of the VON, who argued that the VON was in strong competitive position in relation to for-profits in a market where nurses were in short supply. (Interview with the author, September 1999.)

111 Interview with the author, October 1999. This is a concern also voiced by the associations representing the non-profit and for-profit providers respectively.
112 *Reclaiming a Vision*, 9.
113 See Pat Armstrong and Hugh Armstrong, *Wasting Away*, and Pat Armstrong et al, *Medical Alert*.
114 Interview with the author, September 27, 1999.
115 *Reclaiming a Vision*, 4, 6.
116 "The physical and social conditions in client homes are variable, ranging from excellent (the home is readily amenable to providing appropriate care) to terrible (the home is in poor condition, with inadequate plumbing, poor heating systems or there are family members present who are themselves problematic and sometimes dangerous to workers).

"Home-care work is viewed by some potential workers as lonely and isolating because there are not other colleagues in the home to suggest solutions to problems or to help out in difficult situations. Sometimes home-care workers are working in very challenging situations and must be able to make appropriate decisions on their own." (Margaret MacAdam, *Human Resource Issues in Home Care in Canada*.)
117 Ibid.
118 *The Ottawa Citizen*, June 26, 1998, C8; *The Globe and Mail*, July 6, 1998.
119 *The Ottawa Citizen*, July19, 1998.
120 *The Ottawa Citizen*, October 6, 1998.
121 Chris Hornsey, "Red Cross may lose local office: Agency's homemakers veto a requested cut in their pay," *The Windsor Star*, August 25, 1999.
122 Anne Jarvis, "Red Cross service to shut down: Homemakers worked with sick, frail elderly," *The Windsor Star*, September 15, 1999.
123 Interview with the author, September 1999.
124 *Reclaiming a Vision*, 4.
125 Interview with the author, October 18, 1999.
126 Initially, it was announced that the privately delivered service would cost $830,000 more. This estimate was later revised to half a million dollars.
127 Letter from Monita O'Connor, Acting Regional Director, Long-Term Care Division, Ministry of Health, to Suzanne McGlashan, CEO, Ottawa-Carleton CCAC, May 18, 1999.
128 Quoted by Evelyn Shapiro, *op. cit.*, 9 (emphasis added).
129 It is interesting to see hospitals themselves considering the option of competing for home-care contracts. See *The Hospital-Home Interface:*

Current State and Future Opportunities, Toronto, Ontario Hospital Association, December 1998.

130 According to Peter Coyte and Wendy Young, "the provision of home care rehabilitation services may have resulted in individuals being discharged with home care services 'quicker and sicker' (...) such clients [account] for approximately 40 percent of the annual home-care caseload and 30 percent of total home-care expenditures in Ontario." (Coyte and Young, 4.)

Conclusion

1 Brendan Martin, *In the Public Interest? Privatization and Public Sector Reform*, London, Zed Books, 1993, 84.
2 Ibid., 87. Martin adds: "Having enjoyed growth in public and private sector consultancy income estimated at between 31 per cent in the United States and 47 per cent in Britain over the decade to the late 1980s, income from privatization consultancy alone has doubled every year since then, according to Eric Anstee, who is in charge of international privatization for Ernst & Young. Anstee also revealed the scale of the fortunes being made by a few for devising cost-saving schemes often involving loss of jobs, pay and conditions for many. His own services, and those of other Ernst & Young partners, cost £2,000 (about $3,500) per day. There are some part-time hospital cleaners in Britain who are paid less or little more than that per year for doing more work than they did before consultancy firms like Ernst & Young advised their employers how to achieve value for money. The secret of value for money, it seems, is to pay consultants very well to tell you to pay workers very badly or to get rid of them entirely. Asked if he could understand the reluctance of public sector workers to agree to cost-cutting programs that sacrificed their jobs and services, Eric Anstee replied: 'The only ones who would be against efficiency cuts are the ones who are looking for an easy ride.'" (Ibid., 88.) In the words of Frank Dobson, the Labour Party's energy spokesperson while they were in opposition: "Privatization is a system of outdoor relief for the advisory classes." (Ibid., 90.)
3 "But the fee-for-service system, an ever-increasing number of physicians, a rapidly rising utilization of health-care services, and evidence that physicians and other providers created their own demand, i.e. that patient use of physician services was potentially unlimited and partially directed by physicians' notions of what was a reasonable income, led, step by step, to curbs on medical power. Thus, medicare, from its inception, contained its own political and fiscal

contradictions which led the state, now the guarantor of health services, to rationalize health care. When rising health care costs were met in a number of economic recessions by shrinking government revenues, the stage was set for government-led health care reform and significant state constraints on medical power." (David Coburn and Susan Rappolt, "The 'Logic of Medicare,' Variants of Capitalism and Medical Dominance: Contextualizing Profession-State Relationships," in David Coburn, Susan Rappolt, Ivy Lynn Bourgeault and Jan Angus, *Medicine, Nursing and the State*, 140-141.)

4   Ahmed Bayoumi, "The fine print in the blueprint," *Medical Reform* (Newsletter of the Medical Reform Group), 19:1 (June 1999), 1.
5   Pat Armstrong used this expression in an interview on the local CBC radio station in the Ottawa area on April 10, 2000.
6   Robert Evans, "Health Reform: What 'Business' Is It of Business?" in Daniel Drache and Terry Sullivan, *op. cit.*, 28.
7   Michael Rachlis, *A Review of the Alberta Private Hospital Proposal*, 5.
8   For reviews of these studies, see Michael Rachlis, *op. cit.*, and Kevin Taft and Gillian Steward, *op. cit.*
9   Consumers' Association of Canada (Alberta Branch), "Provincial Consumer Survey on Access to Cataract Surgery Casts Doubt on Claims by Private Health Interests," press release and "Backgrounder," March 1999; and the same organization's information bulletins, "Patient Charges for 'Enhanced' Cataract Lens," and "Waiting Times for Publicly Insured Cataract Surgery," May 1999. See also the study of waiting times for cataract surgery conducted by the Manitoba Centre for Health Policy and Evaluation, "Waiting Times for Surgery in Manitoba," July 1998.
10 Michael Rachlis, *op. cit.*, passim.
11 Robert Evans, "Health Reform: What 'Business' Is It of Business?" 36.
12 See Jim Stanford, "Beware the market madness," *The Globe and Mail*, January 25, 2000.
13 I am grateful to Michelle Weinroth for suggesting this connection.
14 "Peasants have since time immemorial employed various means of regulating land use in the interests of the village community. They have restricted certain practices and granted certain rights, not in order to enhance the wealth of landlords or states but in order to preserve the peasant community itself, perhaps to conserve the land or to distribute its fruits more equitably, and often to provide for the community's less fortunate members. Even private ownership of property has been typically conditioned by such customary practices, giving non-owners certain use rights to property owned by someone else. In England, there were many such practices and cus-

toms. There existed common lands, on which members of the community might have grazing rights or the right to collect firewood, and there were various other kinds of use rights on private land, such as the right to collect the leavings of the harvest during specified periods of the year.

"From the standpoint of improving landlords and capitalist farmers, the land had to be liberated from any such obstruction to their productive and profitable use of property. Between the sixteenth and eighteenth centuries, there was growing pressure to extinguish customary rights that interfered with capitalist accumulation. This could mean various things: disputing communal rights to common lands by claiming exclusive private ownership; eliminating various use rights on private land; or challenging the customary tenures that gave many small-holders rights of possession without unambiguous legal title." (Ellen Meiksins Wood, *The Origin of Capitalism*, New York, Monthly Review Press, 1999, 82.)

[15] Quoted by Ellen Meiksins Wood, *op. cit.*, 83.